Trauma and Intellectual Disability

Acknowledgement, Identification & Intervention

Nigel Beail, Pat Frankish
and Allan Skelly

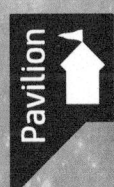

Pavilion

Trauma and Intellectual Disability
Acknowledgment, Identification & Intervention

The authors have asserted their rights in accordance with the Copyright, Designs and Patents Act (1988) to be identified as the authors of this work.

Published by:
Pavilion Publishing and Media Ltd
Blue Sky Offices, 25 Cecil Pashley Way
Shoreham by Sea, West Sussex
BN43 5FF

Tel: 01273 434 943
Email: info@pavpub.com
Web: www.pavpub.com

Published 2021

A catalogue record for this book is available from the British Library.

ISBN: 978-1-914010-59-0

Pavilion Publishing and Media is a leading publisher of books, training materials and digital content in mental health, social care and allied fields. Pavilion and its imprints offer must-have knowledge and innovative learning solutions underpinned by sound research and professional values.

Editors: Nigel Beail, Pat Frankish, Allan Skelly
Production editor: Louisa Robertson, Pavilion Publishing and Media Ltd
Cover design: Emma Dawe, Pavilion Publishing and Media Ltd
Page layout and typesetting: Phil Morash, Pavilion Publishing and Media Ltd
Printing: Severn

Contents

Editor bios

Nigel Beail is a Consultant Clinical Psychologist and Professional Lead for Psychological Services for South West Yorkshire Partnership NHS Foundation Trust, and Professor of Psychology at the Clinical Psychology Unit, Department of Psychology at the University of Sheffield, UK. He is a Fellow of the British Psychological Society (BPS), a Trustee of the British Institute for Learning Disabilities, CPD Lead for the British Psychological Society's DCP Faculty for Learning Disability, former President of European Association for Mental Health in Intellectual Disability, and a founder and Fellow of the Institute for Psychotherapy and Disability. He has published extensively on practice-based research from his clinical work.

Pat Frankish is a Clinical Psychologist and Psychotherapist with many years of experience in the field of disability, emotional development and trauma. Her doctoral study established a method for measuring emotional developmental stages and this has now become the *Frankish Assessment of the Impact of Trauma (FAIT)* published by Pavilion Publishing and Media Ltd (2019). Pat is from Lincolnshire and has settled back there after working in North Yorkshire and Teesside. She has a small group of businesses with her daughter and provides expert psychological services as well as direct support for very distressed individuals in supported living environments. Pat is a past President of the British Psychological Society and has always maintained a strong interest in systemic effects of policy and guidelines. She continues to speak publicly and provide training for staff working at all levels of security and community provisions, including schools. She remains committed to making a difference to the provision she witnessed as a child living with parents who worked in an old long-stay hospital.

Allan Skelly is the 2019–2021 Chair of the Faculty for People with Intellectual Disabilities (FPID) of the British Psychological Society (BPS) and Consultant Clinical Psychologist with Cumbria, Northumberland, Tyne & Wear NHS Foundation Trust. Allan has published articles promoting a focus on the close personal relationships of people with an intellectual disability, the heightened lifetime risk that these will be broken or strained, and how to address this in clinical work. Allan actively promotes the Trauma-Informed Care agenda and the application of Attachment Theory in doing this. He is the author of published articles promoting psychodynamic approaches to people with an intellectual disability, as well as applying Attachment Theory-based interventions in clinical practice. Allan was chair of the working group which produced the 2017 BPS clinical practice guidelines for the integration of Attachment Theory into the work of clinical psychologists in the UK. As well as reviewing the available clinical tools for formal assessment in several publications, he has collaborated on the design and validation of specific tools for this purpose.

Author bios

Sophie Doswell has been working with individuals with learning disability/and or autism for 20 years. She is currently a Consultant Clinical Psychologist for a large London NHS Trust, working with adults with autism and Chair of the Faculty for People with Intellectual Disabilities within the British Psychological Society. Sophie is a passionate advocate of Intensive Interaction and has successfully utilised this approach within a range of settings in

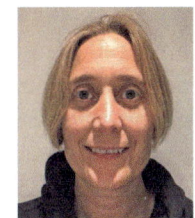

the UK and in long-stay institutions in Serbia and Romania. Sophie and Judith Samuel have previously presented at the British Psychological Society's 'Advancing Practice' conference regarding integrating Intensive Interaction with other approaches.

Elisabeth Goad is a Lead Clinical Psychologist working in Surrey and Borders Partnership NHS Foundation Trust in a Community Team for People with Learning Disabilities. With a special interest in relational approaches and the impact of adverse experiences on people with learning disabilities, developing trauma-informed care within teams has become a life-long passion. Other clinical interests include developing compassion

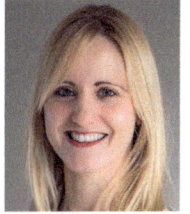

focused interventions for people with learning disabilities and the integration between the theory of compassion and interventions for trauma. Elisabeth is also a guest lecturer at The University of Surrey and enjoys integrating trauma-informed thinking across a range of topics. In her spare time, Elisabeth loves anything that involves being outside in the fresh air, usually alongside family, friends and with a small brown dog in tow.

Cathy Harding has worked as a clinical psychologist for the past 15 years in community, inpatient and supported living services alongside people with an intellectual disability, primarily in South Wales. She actively seeks to ensure that people's histories are integrated into their care and to support and facilitate that people feel empowered in their lives through this approach. This includes supporting people whose behaviours are challenging

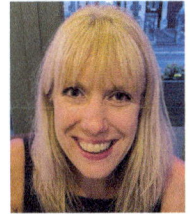

for them, for their staff teams and for their inclusion; due to multifaceted reasons including complex trauma. She offers individual therapy interventions, formulation approaches with individuals and their systems; including supporting staff teams to reflect on their practice, contain and understand distress in its many forms. She also enjoys baking and eating cake and being outside with her family.

Nic Jones works as an independent Consultant Clinical Psychologist, but was previously employed in the NHS for 24 years where she held a few jobs all focusing on neurodiversity (generally, at the same time!). Nic worked in and/or led services dedicated to people on the Autism Spectrum, for those supporting Adults with an Intellectual Disability, and also with children who are fostered or adopted. She is indebted to her clients for sharing their 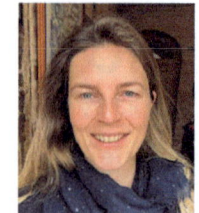 experiences, being willing for those stories to be shared with others and for teaching her along the way. Nic is currently working at The Family Place, a specialist, family-focused Attachment Trauma service on the Welsh-English border. Her work here includes providing a mix of direct therapeutic support, teaching, training and consultation. When away from work Nic is a keen walker, an enthusiastic – though not necessarily informed – gardener, lazy beekeeper, happy cook and novice sailor.

Brett Kahr is Senior Fellow at the Tavistock Institute of Medical Psychology in London, and, also, Visiting Professor of Psychoanalysis and Mental Health in the Regent's School of Psychotherapy and Psychology, at Regent's University London. Additionally, he serves as a Consultant Psychotherapist at The Balint Consultancy and as a Trustee of Freud Museum London. He has maintained a long-standing interest in disability 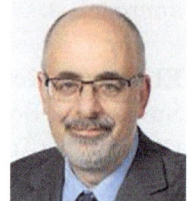 psychotherapy, having worked for many years as Course Tutor in Mental Handicap in the Child and Family Department at the Tavistock Clinic and as a co-founder of the Institute of Psychotherapy and Disability. Likewise, he has also devoted much time to forensic psychotherapy, and works as Consulting Editor to *The International Journal of Forensic Psychotherapy* and serves on the Executive Board of the International Association for Forensic Psychotherapy. Kahr has authored 15 books, including, most recently, *Dangerous Lunatics: Trauma, Criminality, and Forensic Psychotherapy*. His forthcoming book is entitled *Freud's Pandemics: Surviving Global War, Spanish Flu, and the Nazis*.

Judith Samuel is a clinical psychologist with 38 years experience working within health, social care and special educational settings starting as a community psychologist in the East End of London. She has lived and worked in Oxfordshire for the past 28 years. Her clinical work has been mainly with adults and children with ID. Judith's research and service development interests have focused on Intensive Interaction. She became Head of Psychology 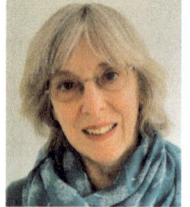 Services for Oxfordshire Learning Disability NHS Trust in 2008. On retirement in 2016, she resumed clinical work in an NHS Learning Disability Community Team. Judith has had a long-standing involvement with the Oxford Doctoral Course in Clinical Psychology and has had two terms of office twenty years apart, as chair of the British Psychological Society, Division of Clinical Psychology, Faculty for people with ID. She is a trustee of FarmAbility: a charity supporting purposeful outdoor activity for co-farmers with ID.

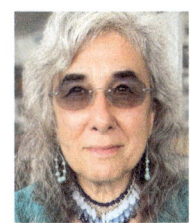

Valerie Sinason is a poet, writer and retired child psychotherapist and adult psychoanalyst who was a consultant at the Tavistock clinic and St. George's Hospital. She has worked for 40 years in the field of intellectual disability and trauma and is President of the Institute for Psychotherapy and Disability (IPD). She has published over 15 books and 160 papers and chapters in the fields of disability, dissociation and trauma. Her key text, 'Mental handicap and the human condition', came out in a revised second edition in 2010. Her latest book, *The Truth about Trauma and Dissociation: everything you didn't want to know and were afraid to ask* (Confer Books, 2020), was awarded the Frank W Putnam Award by the International Society for the Study of Trauma and Dissociation. Her first novel, *The Orpheus Project*, will be published by Aeon Books in 2022.

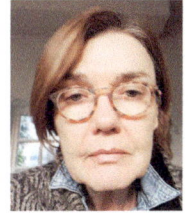

Biza Stenfert Kroese is a Consultant Clinical Psychologist and a Senior Researcher in the School of Psychology at the University of Birmingham, UK, and Chair of *CanDo*, a support service for parents with intellectual disabilities. She is co-author of *Cognitive Behaviour Therapy for People with Intellectual Disabilities: Thinking Creatively* (Palgrave Macmillan 2017). Much of her work is focused on how to adapt psychological assessment and treatment methods to the needs of clients with intellectual disabilities and her research and publications on trauma and talking therapies are informed by her clinical experiences and practice. She is currently a co-investigator for a clinical research trial of EMDR for adults with intellectual disabilities with complex trauma and is chief investigator for a feasibility study on introducing an emotional literacy programme into SEND schools.

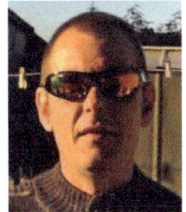

Roger Wilczek has lived with mental health problems since he was 14 years old, and he has a learning disability. He wasn't told this until he was 43. After finally getting help and seeing a psychologist, and getting a few hours a week of support, he learned that he can do something to stop bad treatment of children with learning disabilities, and help them get over it too. He has been an expert by experience since 2016, when he did a talk for all of the health professionals, social care professionals, people with learning disabilities and their families as part of the FPID (Faculty For People With Intellectual Disabilities) Annual Conference in 2021, which built his confidence to speak up. He has written an article and chapter on disability and mental health, and in 2021 he did a talk to the British Psychological Society called "Life Lessons", which was about how important it is to be kind to children with disabilities; love them; give them a good life and not push them aside.

Foreword

Professor Sheila the Baroness Hollins

I thank the editors for inviting me to write a foreword for this important book.

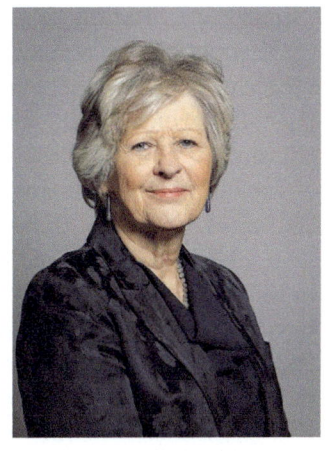

Far too often, the lives of people with intellectual disabilities are subjected to cruelty and neglect. The reality of their own inner worlds, their own hopes and dreams, only briefly connects to public consciousness in news stories and articles, and they are all too readily forgotten in the realm of public policy and health care ethics. For years, we have seen that people have been ignored, maltreated and even left to waste away in the care system. Joan Bicknell, the first female professor of psychiatry in Britain, and my first mentor in my career in intellectual disability psychiatry, had championed the introduction of family-style care in the late 1970s. She called for multi-disciplinary approaches to developing community alternatives to mental handicap hospitals which were under the control of medical superintendents. Such places were replete with impersonal care, neglect or worse. For those who were cared for by their families, Joan also reminded us of the adjustment families had to make in the face of the news that their child would have a different life path than the one expected (Bicknell, 1983).

Institutional care of the kind seen in the mental handicap hospitals has now mostly gone, partly thanks to Joan's leadership in kickstarting the modernisation of care in a task force appointed to address the scandal of Normansfield Hospital in 1978. However, we still see disturbing, familiar features of sadistic 'care' such as at Winterbourne View in 2011, and more recently at Whorlton Hall and Muckamore Abbey. It has never been easy to establish basic human rights for people with intellectual disabilities following decades of institutionalisation. While progress has been made, in far too many places, aspirations for a well-supported ordinary life remain low and there is still a very long way to go. In the UK in 2021, several thousand people are in hospital receiving care or containment from clinical teams on hospital wards detained under mental health legislation. Their care seldom includes any therapeutic purpose and individual outcomes are poor. This is at least partly because the community facilities that would be safe enough to live in, and create the feeling of family that Joan Bicknell championed, have not been properly funded and developed (Wood, 2020).

Writing in the British Journal of Psychiatry, Valerie Sinason and I drew attention to the lack of consideration given to the trauma visited upon people with intellectual disabilities, and the rarity of any psychological therapies being offered to help them (Sinason and Hollins, 2000). Soon afterwards, the Royal College of Psychiatrists (RCP) published *Psychotherapy and Learning Disability* (2004), the first document with clear survey evidence on the therapeutic offer available in the UK. More than 420 professionals who were offering psychological therapies responded to the survey, and despite a limited evidence base either for or against therapeutic efficacy, and lack of inclusion or equal access to mainstream psychological therapies, they were upbeat about their own therapeutic work. The range of therapies have continued to develop since then, with incremental improvements in research evidence, including from controlled trials (Beail, 2016). The idea that psychotherapy will not work with this group is turning out to be unfounded, and the family of psychotherapies proliferate. While much of this therapy is primarily focused on symptoms of anxiety, depression, anger, self-esteem etc., this often also addresses earlier abuse (Sequeira and Hollins, 2003). We now know that people with intellectual disabilities are much more likely to be maltreated, thanks to well-conducted epidemiological studies in several countries, with a large scale study in the UK being completed in Sussex in 2005 (Spencer *et al.*, 2005).

At the end of the last decade, it seems that the same human need for deep and enduring emotional attachments across the lifespan came into frame for people with disabilities, as for others (Fletcher *et al.*, 2016; British Psychological Society, 2017). None too soon. Rapid changes of living circumstances, widespread use of agency care staff, underfunded care, multiple placement, a focus on 'coping skills' rather than relationship stability, the trauma of admission to hospital, and naïve models of independent living, are all practices that are being challenged by attachment theory literature. This is welcome, because the comfort and security of close relationship bonds contain the conditions required for healing, especially for trauma caused by sexual, emotional and physical abuse in childhood. It requires a commitment to substantial human interaction to establish this sense of psychological safety that will eventually allow them to grow and enjoy their lives. Care and intervention should reflect the level of need, and not be unnecessarily brief, inaccessible, or impersonal in nature. We need to give something of ourselves in this endeavour.

The organisation I established after my retirement has these objectives at its heart. Books Beyond Words creates stories about relationships, including stories about trauma and healing and aims to empower people trying to live their lives outside 'service-land' as well as people who are recipients of services (https://booksbeyondwords.co.uk).

This book brings together a long but neglected tradition. The messages of acknowledgment, identification, and intervention speaks to past denials at all levels of society. The book gives an historical perspective, personal accounts, figures and data, the theory to explain, and models of treatment.

No reason remains to fail in addressing trauma in the lives of people with intellectual disabilities. The contributors to this book have dedicated their work to that purpose. I endorse and commend it to the reader, and I am sure it will find a wide audience.

References

Beail N (2016) *Psychological therapies and people who have Intellectual disabilities: a report from the Royal College of Psychiatrists and British Psychological Society*. Leicester: British Psychological Society.

Bicknell J (1983). The psychopathology of handicap. *British Journal of Medical Psychology* **56** (2) 167-78.

British Psychological Society (2017) *Incorporating Attachment Theory into Practice: Clinical Practice Guideline for Clinical Psychologists working with People who have Intellectual Disabilities*. Leicester, UK: British Psychological Society.

Fletcher H, Flood A & Hare D (2016) *Attachment in Intellectual and Developmental Disability: A Clinician's Guide to Practice and Research*. New York: Wiley.

Royal College of Psychiatrists (2004) *Psychotherapy and Learning Disability*. Council Report CR116: London: Royal College of Psychiatrists.

Sequeira, H & Hollins S (2003) Clinical effects of sexual abuse on people with learning disability. *British Journal of Psychiatry*, **182** 13-19.

Sinason V & Hollins S (2000) Psychotherapy, learning disabilities and trauma: new perspectives. *The British Journal of Psychiatry*, **176** (1) 32-36.

Spencer N, Devereux E, Wallace A, Sundrum R, Shenoy M, Bacchus C & Logan S (2005) Disabling conditions and registration for child abuse and neglect: A population-based study. *Paediatrics* **116** (3) 609–14.

Wood A (2020) Helping People Thrive. https://www.learningdisabilityengland.org.uk/wp-content/uploads/2020/06/Helping-People-Thrive-00000002.pdf

Chapter 1: Introduction to Trauma and Intellectual Disability: why this book is needed

Nigel Beail

This book is about trauma-informed care (TIC) for people who have intellectual disabilities (ID). The history of abuse against people who have ID is documented in Chapters 2 and 3, as well as the recognition that this continues in some residential services and in our communities. While such abuse has become well known and documented, the acknowledgement and identification that this causes trauma has come much later to the table. It has taken a long time for professionals and service providers to accept that such experiences, along with other adverse childhood and life experiences, may have negative outcomes in that they traumatise people. The recognition of the need to address trauma emerged in psychotherapeutic work in the 1980s (see Chapter 4), but the acceptance of TIC in services for people who have ID is much more recent. TIC emerged into more widespread consciousness among health professions in the early 2000s, initially in the United States in services for the adult general population who had mental health concerns (Harris and Fallott, 2001; Jennings, 2004), and then in children's services (Hodas, 2006). However, despite trauma being recognised by a small group of people developing psychological therapies for people who have ID (Chapter 4), it was not until a decade later that the new service philosophy started to be seen as relevant in services for people who have ID.

What is trauma?

The term 'trauma' is widely used, but a helpful standard definition is "an event, a series of events or a set of circumstances that is experienced by an individual as physically or emotionally harmful or life-threatening." (SAMHSA, 2014). Due to the evidence of the differential impact of short-term, one-off, and long-term, repeated traumatic events, Terr (1991) has devised a commonly used categorisation:

- Type 1 trauma: sudden and unexpected events experienced as isolated incidents, such as road traffic accidents, rapes or terrorist attacks. These can happen in childhood or adulthood.

- Type 2 trauma: repeated or ongoing traumatic events, such as generally happens in the abuse of children and adults who have ID e.g. physical, emotional and sexual abuse, and sexual exploitation. In recent years this has, by convention, been referred to as 'complex trauma'.

Such traumatic events or circumstances are experienced by an individual as physically or emotionally harmful, or life-threatening, and this results in adverse effects on the individual's psychological functioning and well-being. This extends to actual reductions in brain volume (e.g. Bremner, 2006) and so trauma can be argued to alter the very essence of who one is, and how one acts. Trauma can affect people at any time in their life, but some sectors of the population are more vulnerable. Research on traumatic or adverse childhood experiences (ACEs) show that these are strong risk factors for negative physical and mental health outcomes for people who have ID and the more ACEs one has, the higher the risk (Catani and Sossalla, 2015). People who have ID are also at risk of experiencing more adverse life experiences (ADLs) too (Emerson and Brigham, 2014) as they go through life.

Trauma- and stress-related disorders are included in the American Psychiatric Association's Diagnostic and Statistical Manual-5 (APA, 2013) and its companion manual DM-ID 2 for people who have ID (Fletcher, Barnhill and Cooper, 2016). In the chapter on trauma- and stress-related disorders, McCathy *et al.* (2016) examine the five classifications for different types of trauma presentation listed in DSM-5, and how they may manifest in people who have ID. These are reactive attachment disorder (RAD), disinhibited engagement disorder (DED), post-traumatic stress disorder (PTSD), acute stress disorder, and adjustment disorders. With RAD, McCarthy, *et al.* (2016) suggest that considering the person's actual attachment behaviours, and addressing these, may be more fruitful (and scientific) than taking a diagnostic approach. DED is also believed to result from disrupted attachment, but there is limited evidence regarding the validity of this diagnosis with people who have ID. This is also the case for acute stress disorder and adjustment disorders. For PTSD, McCarthy, *et al.* (2016) report that for people with mild ID the presentation is the same as that for the general population. This includes symptoms of recurrent, involuntary intrusive memories, recurrent distressing dreams, dissociation, and intense and prolonged psychological distress. People who have PTSD may also try to avoid distressing thoughts, feeling and memories, and experience marked alterations in their thoughts, mood, bodily arousal and reactivity when reminded of the circumstances of the trauma. For people who have more severe IDs, one might expect that trauma may be noticed via behavioural symptoms, such as trauma specific re-enactments, simply because they are less able to express their feelings using spoken language (e.g. over-reacting to changes in their caregivers; seeking to interact in an anxious manner; asking for direction more than required; becoming hostile in response to minor frustrations, responding to new caregivers with unnecessary fear, etc.). In the experience of the editors of this book, we see a wide range of signs and symptoms of psychological distress communicated verbally, or through behaviour for people of all levels of ID. As illustrated in Chapter 11 that which cannot be spoken will be acted out.

This book refers to the urgency of the need for greater trauma-informed working with people who have an ID. Being trauma-informed means an individual being aware that the psychological, emotional and/or behavioural difficulties a person they are supporting, providing services for or providing treatment for, may have experienced trauma in their life. Further, being trauma-informed means understanding how trauma affects the person and knowing effective ways to respond to someone who has experienced it (Marcal and Trifoso 2017). A key message is that everyone has a role to play in recognising, preventing, understanding and responding to the trauma commonly experienced by people whose disability creates challenges in and of itself. We all need to relate to people we encounter using trauma-informed principles, regardless of whether a history of trauma is known or identified. All people who work with people who have ID need to be able to identify the types of experiences that are traumatic and identify situations that can bring back memories of trauma and associated feelings. All staff need the basic competencies of being able to listen and empathically engage with the people they work with. Using the British Psychological Society's Power Threat Meaning Framework (Johnstone *et al.*, 2018), we need to ask people 'What has happened to you?' instead of 'What is wrong with you?' This approach also asked how the trauma affected the person, what sense they make of it and what they did to survive. However, this approach was developed with adults in the general population and I have found that it needs some adaptation when used with people who have ID. For example, when working with a young man who experienced abuse for years, he could not say what had happened to him. To survive, he kept such memories out of conscious thought or warded them off. However, through a period of exploratory psychotherapy he began to be able to access those memories and start to tell me what happened to him. The impact on him was clear during our exploration as he showed considerable distress. Gradually, over time, he was able to see what meaning his experiences had for him and see that what are called maladaptive behaviours or behaviours that challenge were his means of survival.

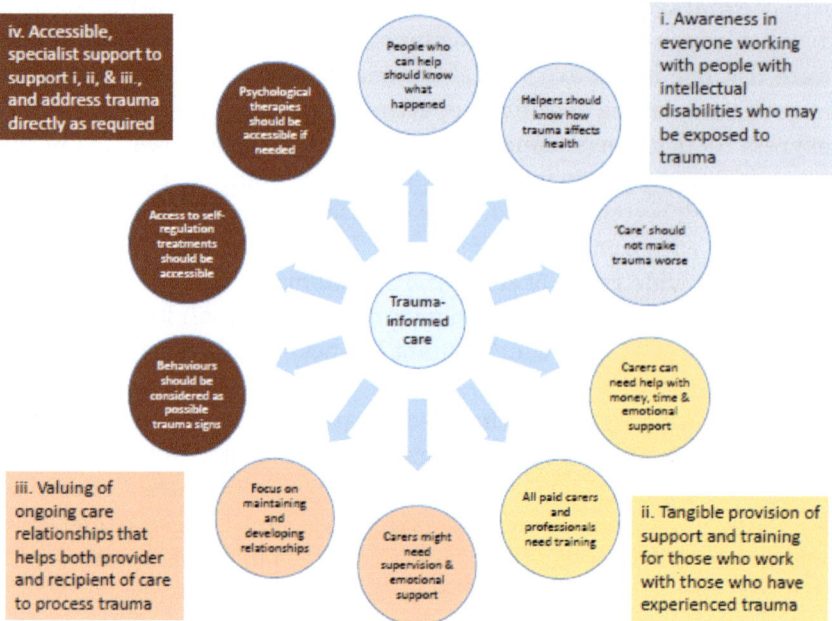

Figure 1.1: The Learning Disability Professional Senate 10 Top Tips for TIC (reproduced by kind permission)

Families and health- and care-staff who support people who have an ID and have experienced trauma also need to be aware of TIC. The Learning Disability Senate (2020) has developed a poster for families and health- and care-staff who work with people who have an ID. The poster contains 10 top tips on the trauma-informed approach to people who have ID (see Figure 1.1). The 10 tips are broken into four areas of increasing levels of knowledge and skill: awareness; training and support; specialised support in dealing with trauma; and direct specialist interventions. The senate asks that all carers and professionals are trauma-aware and understand its impact on the person's health and well-being. They point out that people who have ID are more at risk of trauma than those in the general population, and as such may need greater support. They recognise that change at any stage of life can be traumatising. They argue that families should have the resources and support they need to develop positive attachments with their child. The senate has gone as far as to say that care staff and professionals need compulsory training in TIC to improve their awareness, understanding and skills in preventing exposure to trauma, and supporting those who have been traumatised. Additionally, families and care staff need support and time to reflect, so that they feel valued and can respond in ways that make people feel safe. Supporters also need to know the person they support well and know their trauma history, and that this is incorporated into any support plan. Further, support plans should help the person feel safe, have positive relationships, good experiences, control and choice. They state that behaviours should be considered from a trauma perspective, and to imagine, or 'mentalise' the person's experiences, rather than thinking of them in terms of the behaviours that are observed. This might mean addressing language used about a person such as 'having a behaviour', becoming something more akin to 'having an experience'. The senate also states that people who have ID and have been traumatised should have access to specialist services and appropriate therapies that have been adjusted to meet their needs.

In this book, we want to promote the acknowledgement, identification of trauma in the lives of people who have ID and then the means of intervention. A helpful model guiding our aims is that of Herman (1992). He has put forward a phased based model of trauma and recovery. In the model, it is stated that interventions for the effects of trauma should aim to promote physical safety and coping with the impact of trauma, enhance emotional stability, reduce emotional distress linked to the memory of past trauma and enable the person to make active life choices. So, people who have ID should have access to early and rigorous assessments so that trauma is safely recognised and understood, and its immediate effects addressed at the earliest possible opportunity so that people can be protected from ongoing or future harm. People who have been affected by trauma should be enabled to develop effective coping strategies to help them manage their lives, both current and past, and to develop safe and nurturing relationships. The model also proposes that people who have been affected by trauma need opportunities to process and make sense of trauma, and be enabled to work through the distress they feel in connection with these events. Lastly, people should be enabled to develop skills, move towards goals and participate in valued roles and experiences that may not have previously been possible, due to trauma.

Thus, people who have ID need to be supported by services that are trauma-aware and informed, and may also need a more specialist response, such as a trauma-informed positive behavioural support plan, as well as one-to-one psychological therapy. It is important to emphasise that not everyone will necessarily need every intervention element of the phased model, and that people can move in both directions through the phases and may spend differing amounts of time in different phases, depending on their current life circumstances and their recovery pathway.

Workforce competencies

Marcel and Trifoso (2017) have produced a trauma-informed toolkit to integrate some of the best practices that can be applied to the work done with people with ID who have experienced trauma. The focus of the toolkit is on areas other than one-to-one interventions, such as psychotherapy, although the principles and information they provide are equally important for therapists to know. Marcel and Trifoso argue that self-care for direct support staff and professionals serving people with trauma is critical, as it positively impacts on the quality of care they provide, and reduces restrictive practices and staff turnover. They provide guidance on trauma-informed behavioural planning and argue that behaviour due to a trauma history potentially needs different interventions. In the assessment phase, Marcel and Trifoso state that the usual functional analysis approach may not find a function or purpose for the behaviour, but such behaviours need understanding. Finally, they offer direction for planning for agency administrators, quality-assurance staff, and interested others. Agencies serving people with IDs are responsible for: minimising restrictive interventions such as physical restraints; interviewing victims of possible abuse; providing training to staff, sensitising them to trauma-related care needs; and overseeing the care provided by direct-support professionals and clinicians.

The National Health Service Education for Scotland (2018), in partnership with the Scottish Government, has developed trauma skilled practice levels. Four levels of knowledge and skills are outlined that are required by all workers who have direct and/or substantial contact with children and adults who may be affected by known or unknown trauma. These levels are all mapped on to the phased model of trauma and recovery (Herman, 1992). These are aimed at the workforce. However, families and all carers in the lives of people who have ID need awareness at a level appropriate to the level of support they are providing.

The trauma-informed practice level describes the baseline knowledge and skills that are required by everyone in the workforce. These knowledge and skills should also be shared with families and informal carers of people who have ID. The trauma skilled practice level describes the knowledge and skills required by all workers who have direct and/or substantial contact with individuals (children and adults) who may be affected by traumatic events, whether or not trauma is known about. This level is likely to be relevant to staff from statutory services, such as health and social care, justice staff, emergency services and third sector-organisations.

Those professionals who provide support or interventions or manage services that have regular and intense contact with those known to be affected by trauma should have an enhanced level of practice. Then there is a specialist level for those professionals who play a specialist role in directly providing:

- evidence-based psychological interventions or therapies to individuals affected by traumatic events, and/or
- in offering consultation to inform the care and treatment, or in managing trauma-specific services, and/or
- in leading on the development of trauma-specific services, and/or
- in co-ordinating multi-agency service-level responses to trauma.

The knowledge and skills outlined at each level of the framework are constructed in an incremental way meaning that, for example, staff operating at the trauma-enhanced practice level would also be expected to possess the knowledge and skills described at the trauma-informed and skilled practice level. The framework does not aim to specify which staff roles correspond to which practice level. Instead, the expectation is that workers and their employers will take responsibility for ensuring that they relevantly interpret and apply the content and aspirations of the framework.

Vicarious trauma

It also needs to be recognised that working with and supporting victims of trauma can have a profound impact on those supporting them; this includes partners, relatives, neighbours and social- and health-care workers. Working with trauma victims may cause profound psychological effects that can become disruptive and painful, and can persist for months or years (McCann and Pearlman, 1990). Our thoughts and emotions, conscious and unconscious, can be negatively transformed through the typical process of empathic engagement with the traumatic accounts of our clients or relatives. The continued exposure to the darkest aspects of the human condition can produce symptoms strikingly akin to post-traumatic symptoms in the people we are working with and supporting (Blair and Ramones, 1996). This process, vicarious traumatisation, and the risk of it occurring in staff and family members, means that all staff and family carers need access to support and supervision to talk about their feelings and reactions to their client's trauma.

In this book we start with an acknowledgement of trauma in the lives of people who have ID with a personal account from an expert by experience (Chapter 2), then an historical overview (Chapter 3), and then the beginnings of recognition in the 1980s (Chapter 4). Chapters 5 and 6 focus on the identification of trauma in the lives of people who have ID. In Chapter 7, we are shown what a trauma-informed service can look like. We then turn to interventions and have tried to cover as many as possible (Chapters 8 to 14), but we are aware this is not comprehensive. We are pleased to cover such a diverse range, including positive behavioural support, intensive interaction, cognitive behavioural therapy (CBT) and eye movement desensitisation and reprocessing, dyadic interpersonal psychotherapy, and developmental and psychodynamic approaches. The range of interventions available to people who have ID is continuously growing. This became very clear when the psychological therapies for people who have ID guidance was revised in 2016 (Beail, 2016). We hope that those providing psychological interventions will continue to take a trauma informed approach.

References

American Psychiatric Association (2013) *Diagnostic and Statistical Manual of Mental Disorders* (5th edition). Arlington, VA: American Psychiatric Publishing.

Beail N (2016) *Psychological Therapies and People who have Intellectual Disabilities*. Leicester: British Psychological Society.

Blair DT & Ramones VA (1996) Understanding vicarious traumatization. *Journal of Psychosocial Nursing Mental Health Services* **34** (11) 2430

Boris NW, Zeanah CH, Larrieu JA, Scheeringa, MS & Heller, SS (1998) Attachment disorders in infancy and early childhood: a preliminary investigation of diagnostic criteria. *American Journal of Psychiatry* **155** 2 295-297.

Bremner JD (2006) Traumatic stress: effects on the brain. *Dialogues in Clinical Neuroscience* **8**(4) 445–461.

Catani C & Sossalla IM (2015) Child abuse predicts adult PTSD symptoms among individuals diagnosed with intellectual disability. *Frontiers in Psychology* **6**, 1-11.

Emerson, E & Brigham, P (2014) Exposure of children with developmental delay to social determinants of poor health: cross-sectional case record review study. *Child: Care, Health and Development* **41**(2), 249-257.

Fletcher R, Barnhill J & Cooper S-A (2016) *Diagnostic Manual – Intellectual Disability Second Edition*. New York: NADD Press.

Harris M & Fallott R (2001) *Using trauma theory to design service systems: New Directions in Mental Health Services 89*. San Francisco: Jossey Bass.

Herman J (1992) *Trauma and Recovery: The Aftermath of Violence— From Domestic Abuse to Political Terror*. New York: Basic Books.

Hodas GR (2006) *Responding to Childhood Trauma: The promise and practice of trauma informed care*. Harrisburg, PA: Pennsylvania Office of Mental Health and Substance Misuse Services.

Jennings A (2004) *Models for Developing Trauma Informed behavioural Health Systems and Trauma Specific Services*. National Association for State Mental Health Services.

Johnstone, L, Boyle, M, with Cromby, J, Dillon, J, Harper, D, Kinderman, P, Longden, E, Pilgrim, D & Read, J (2018) *The Power Threat Meaning Framework: Towards the Identification of Patterns in Emotional Distress, Unusual Experiences and Troubled or Troubling Behaviour, as an Alternative to Functional Psychiatric Diagnosis*. Leicester: British Psychological Society.

Kliewer-Neumann JD, Zimmermann J, Bovenschen I, Gabler S, Lang K, Spangler G & Nowacki K (2018) Assessment of attachment disorder symptoms in foster children: Comparing diagnostic assessment tools. *Child and Adolescent Psychiatry and Mental Health* **12** 43.

Learning Disability Professional Senate (2019) *Top 10 Tips: Trauma Informed Approaches for People who have ID*. London: Learning Disability Professional Senate.

McCann IL & Pearlman LA (1990) *Vicarious traumatisation: A framework for understanding the psychological effects of working with victims. Journal of Traumatic Stress* **3** (1) 131-149.

McCarthy J, Blanco RA Gaus VL Razza NJ & Tomasulo DJ (2016) Trauma- and stress-related disorders. In: R Fletcher, J Barnhill & S-A Cooper, *Diagnostic Manual – Intellectual Disability* (2nd edition). New York: NADD Press.

Marcal S & Trifoso S (2017) *A Trauma-Informed Toolkit for Providers in the Field of Intellectual Disabilities*. New York: Centre for Disability Services.

National Health Service Education for Scotland (2017) *Transforming Psychological Trauma*. Edinburgh: NHS Education for Scotland (on line) available at www.nes.scot.nhs.uk

Substance Abuse and Mental Health Service Administration (2014a). *SAMHSA's concept of trauma and guidance for a trauma-informed approach*. HHS Publication No. (SMA) 14-4884. Rockville, MD: Substance Abuse and Mental Health Services Administration.

Terr, LC (1991) Childhood trauma: An outline and overview. *American Journal of Psychiatry* **148** (1) 10-20.

Chapter 2:
Please stop people going through what I went through – and am still going through

Roger Wilczek

My name is Roger. Apparently, I've had mental health issues since I was 14. I had a learning disability but no one told me. When I was a baby, they did look after me but I was very ill. I was one of four. When I was six months, I went into a fit and doctors turned around to my mum and said: 'If you want to see him for the last time, now's the time.' Not once, but twice. I had bad constipation problems too. And my thought patterns were affected. I owe my life to those doctors and nurses. I heard that when I walked, they said it was a miracle. They didn't expect me to recover because my body was stiff as a table.

When I was a little boy, some bad things happened. Some were little things like people turning their back on me, or they'd stop listening to me when I talked. Some were serious, like having a scraper thrown at me and when my eye was nearly gouged out. And also being locked in a dark place. Sometimes I thought that people hated me or that I shouldn't have lived. There is still some bad blood because of this.

Other times I got beat up so bad that I thought I was going to die. But I got hit a lot of times too. Often on the back of the neck. A lot of the time I couldn't work out why. In northeast England people say 'getting wrong' to mean in trouble. But I didn't know what I had done wrong. I still hate people touching me on the neck. Someone did it when I was a bit older and I punched them. I felt terrible about it because he didn't know I hated it. I would get the blame for things I know I hadn't done. It was easy for other kids to give me the blame because of my disability. I'm not saying I wasn't naughty sometimes, but I couldn't explain very well when it wasn't my fault.

Some of these things are so bad I still get nightmares about them. I would like to say who did them but I've been told I cannot say more in this book because of legal reasons. Anyway, it would be hard to prove now. They might say I made it up or made it sound a lot worse than it was. But I know my mental health came from it because it goes round and round in my head much more when I get depressed or want to kill myself. Memories go together with remembering the bad things that happened, and that goes together with feeling worried, depressed or suicidal. I still get a frightened feeling that goes back to then, when I am worried about something now. Like if they change my benefits or if someone argues with me. That can trigger it off you see. Like the gun is loaded and then the new thing fires it.

Another thing is I would have liked a bit more attention. I would have liked more cuddles but it only happened sometimes with some people. There are some people who were always kind and they really helped me. But some of these guys I don't see any more or hardly ever, or they have died. Actually, I have had a lot of grief in my life. This still rips me apart.

At school I was bullied. They would trip me up, laugh when I hurt myself and call me all sorts; beat me up a few times. I didn't have as much money as the other kids but if you did have any, the bully would steal it. One day when I was fifteen, I sort of snapped and picked on the biggest bully in the school and beat him up. They called my mam in, but she asked them, what do they expect if I get bullied? I never got bullied after that. This taught me to be hard but I don't want to be hard. I am not hard. It was an act I had to do.

The teachers turned a blind eye. They weren't really any help. I heard one of them talk to another saying: 'These kids are not going to make it in life, not going to learn, so there's no point in learning them.' Funny how you remember things that make you feel bad.

I left school at fifteen. With all that went on, it was hard to trust people. Women and men used to rob me. One person got a loan out in my name. When they got caught, they showed me the signature and it wasn't mine. I said: 'Of course it's not.' And you know what? The bank had the cheek to offer me a loan! I couldn't believe it.

In the 1990s, I went clubbing a lot. I had friends and girlfriends. But there were a lot of fights. Because of the way I was they thought they could treat me like crap. They used to call me 'dipshit'. They'd say: 'Dipshit won't know, don't ask him.'

Sometimes I got into scrapes. Once I was bundled into a car and robbed. I thought they might kill me but they just dumped me in the middle of nowhere.

All the time I got called 'Spacca' – a northeast word [UK] that means 'Spastic'. It means you're thick. You're worthless. Everyone was making me out to be a loser and I believed them.

There were some nice moments, like when a girlfriend found out what I had went through as a baby and she just gave me a hug and a kiss and called me her 'miracle boyfriend'. I have had some relationships and was with a really lovely person for several years. It's really sad but she was not well with a serious condition. We tried to carry on but it affected her more and more and she went back to her family. Again, there are some things that I cannot put down on paper that were really awful – they were no one's fault, it was just bad luck. I was devastated to lose her. That's when I started to think I was 100% a loser.

In 2010, my dad passed away. You see, he had cancer but it wasn't diagnosed early enough. So then I didn't trust doctors. I get very worried about aches and pains and I always think it's cancer. If they tell me it's not, I don't believe them. I always think it's cancer. You can get it any time and not know until it's too late. Many of my family have died from it. Some of my friends too.

Of the people who are still alive, there are some that I'd like to see more of. Some folk don't want to talk about the past, they don't like to. It can make them angry or feel like they are getting wrong off me. Some of them have their own illnesses. They see I'm not physically sick and they have a point that they might be worse off in some ways. I understand that and I feel sorry for them. But whatever the reason is, I often end up sitting in my flat on my own and not really seeing anyone and hardly hearing from anyone. All I would like is a little call. A little of their time, not their money or presents or anything. What I want doesn't cost money. I feel like the black sheep.

Looking back on it, there's been a lot of illness among family and friends. A friend died of cancer too. Recently, when two people I cared about died, I wasn't invited to the funerals. It might have been because of coronavirus but I know the first one was before coronavirus. I sometimes wonder was it because I am not wanted there?

Anyway, when I turned forty, social services came in. I was going to commit suicide or starve. My family doctor started to think about the right help for me. He has been really good because when one of my family was really ill, he did right by them, and actually visited the hospital. He's been better than other professionals. Do you know, you can't have a family doctor now? The link with one person is gone. You just get who's 'on' today. One time, someone who didn't know me said: 'it's all in your head.' But they didn't mean I needed to talk to someone or get mental health help. They meant I was making it up. That's horrible.

I smoke a lot because of my depression. My psychologist went with me to see the Stop Smoking nurse. My blood was loaded with bad stuff from smoking. I need to stop for my health. I need to do this soon.

What help have I had, you ask?

I had nothing when I was a kid. I was told to get on with it. Until I was thirty-three, I got nothing. When I was thirty, I met a professional who said: 'I don't trust you.' So, I thought: 'Sod you, pal.' When I was thirty-three, my GP gave me medication. It was the first time my mental health was talked about. But I didn't get my learning disability assessed until I was forty-four, when the community team found out about me from my GP, and someone thought: 'We need to test him.' I should have asked to talk to someone then but I didn't know what I needed.

The treatment I needed was the therapy for depression that I got when I was forty-seven. Forty-seven years old. Therapy has been helping me understand my life and my past. Now I know I'm worth something. My voice does count. I believe this a bit now, but I still feel like a loser a lot of the time. I still feel lonely. But I feel like I wouldn't be here if it wasn't for my psychologist and Mencap. Mencap are there for my physical health and to help me look after myself. They are company for a few hours a week. Therapy has helped me in ways I couldn't imagine.

Why did I have to wait until I was forty-seven? Why did no one check me out? I used to think that if I got ill in my body or my head I wouldn't go to hospital because I'm a loser. I didn't deserve any help. Now I think my psychologist has a point – I do deserve it. Like if I think about a little boy, like I was, if I saw them in need, I'd be there in a shot. Get the bullies off them, give them love. I am like this when I see my sister's grandkids – they give me cuddles. It's lovely. Therapy says 'when you were a little boy, you were lovely too'. It's so hard for me to believe that. To say to yourself with feeling. But now I see it is true. It's like having one guy on your shoulder saying, 'you're a loser' and one guy on your other shoulder saying, 'no way are you a loser'. Like when I do a talk or write something – I can't be a loser then.

I've got to say something about my Mencap staff. I got them after my learning disability diagnosis. They help me read letters, meals and cooking, company. Like Rachel. She has been fantastic even with the coronavirus. We go shopping and I have company and good advice. And they back the therapy up. I am worth something. Rachel's right about most things. Like giving up smoking. So, I'm going to do it, I'm going to get a vape. Also, there's Leanne – with Rachel she has been my rock. Not everyone in my life is like this. Also, there is Jeff. He has a disability too and he understands disability. He is thoughtful. And has a lovely guide dog. I think that they are part of my family.

Why am I writing this down? Here's what I think needs done.

- People need to be kind to children with disabilities. A little bit more care and protection. Children with disabilities need a little more. Don't push a little one away when they're naughty or ask for attention. That's how we get mental health problems; because we think: 'No one loves me and I'm lonely.'

- Give children good beliefs. Don't let children think that they aren't worth anything. Prevention is better than cure.

- Treat mental health as soon as possible. Help children, don't let them struggle by themselves.

- Give us enough to live on. Cuts to our money are frightening. It makes you feel like a loser who doesn't deserve anything. Doesn't deserve to live. Stop it, stop putting the cost of things up, and our money down.

- Support the places that help us. I go to a place called Guidepost, where I feel safe and I feel accepted.

- Don't be afraid to get help for a long time. They might offer you therapy for a short time. But some people need longer. Ask for more therapy if you need it. I needed longer, I needed years because of what happened to me. I became an Expert by Experience. So, in a way, this is 'therapy plus'. It makes me feel good to help others, like doing this chapter. I heard that someone spoke up about what happened to her, because of a talk I did. That brought me to tears. Good tears.

- Help more people like me speak up. Why doesn't the Government ever talk about us on the TV? What do they decide? It really matters because it changes things like our money. We're left in the dark. They cut your money or say you can't get a service you used to get. It feels like there's nothing you can do about it.

The last thing I want to say: please listen to me and people like me. If people can't talk, find out about them and help them. Don't say 'you're a number on a card' or treat us like cattle. Every one of them numbers on the card is a person with a story and a life to lead. Our voice should count.

Editor's note:

This chapter is based on an edited transcription of an interview, edited by Roger in further discussions with Allan Skelly. To help Roger with structuring his recall, the following prompts were used at various points in the interview:

- *Let's start with what happened to you as a baby…*
- *What happened when you were a little boy at home…*
- *What was school like…?*
- *After school, how did you get on…?*
- *Tell me about your long-term relationship.*
- *Tell me about the help you've had in your life.*
- *What needs to happen in your opinion?*

Some text has been edited on advice from the publisher with Roger's approval.
AS

Chapter 3:
The history of disability is a history of trauma

Valerie Sinason

We are all walking history. To be alive now means we have had ancestors who experienced unknown dangers and pleasures in every period of history. Items over 50 years are called vintage and over 100 years are antiques. What does that mean over the huge weight of history we all carry? Some aspects of our personality and appearance and behaviour could go back not just to grandparents and great-grandparents, but even further. Carrying the history of our ancestors can be light or heavy. Some ways we carry history can be surprising. One aristocrat, who could trace his family back to the Norman conquest of 1066, told me he woke up in a bedroom decorated by his ancestors and walked down the stairs for breakfast passing full-length paintings of them. They looked like him and because he came from a known family, whose family histories were recorded, the terrible endings some of them met – killed in battle, poisoned, strangled, executed – were also known. At the other end of the scale was an orphan, a former child refugee from the Middle East who did not know anything of her family history. She was a vibrant and successful human being. 'I have no history weighing me down. There is just me. I am lucky to be alive. I can make my own history.' Where did that resilience come from?

Sometimes our history, known or unknown, is linked to our personality, nationality, religion, or the colour of our hair and eyes. Sometimes it is genetically linked to our ability and disability. What does it feel like to carry a history that is linked to disability? How does that affect your identity and sense of culture? Anna (not her real name), who had Down's syndrome, said she saw someone on a school outing who looked just like her. She went to her local school after her loving parents fought successfully for her inclusion. However, she felt a deep sense of loss; there was no one she considered like her there. On the school trip, they joined up with other schools and the brief sight of another girl with Down's syndrome made her feel she had found her missing family.

In a London school filled with children whose parents or grandparents had come from Syria, Afghanistan, the Yemen, there were pieces of pain and yearning in their minds. They were exiles from a long and troubled and proud history. Anna did not have a country she was in exile from. That was her terrible sense of loss. There is not a Down's syndrome country, a cerebral palsy country. There are only the fluctuating, historical waves of inclusion and exclusion, of fear, of pity, of hate. The disability or handicap or difficulty, whatever historical name is in use, has its own history. We can trace the treatment and experience of disability as far back as human history goes. But there is a truncated feeling often in the individual that they have been crossed off their family tree.

When I worked at the London hospital over 40 years ago, there was fear in different minorities at registering births because of the international shame it would cause, or the difficulty it would cause in arranging to marry-off other children because of genetic concerns. The wish to 'write-off' from history the family member with an intellectual disability (ID) has always been known. Nerissa and Katherine Bowes-Lyon – nieces of the Queen Mother were cousins to Queen Elizabeth II and had been kept since 1941 in the Royal Earlswood Asylum for Mental Defectives in Surrey. Edward VII expressed relief when his autistic brother, who also suffered from epilepsy, died and called him 'more of an animal'. And of course, at the same time, we have, around the world, examples of loving inclusion. However, a look at the history of disability mainly reveals the shadow side of human behaviour.

What is the deepest, most worrying fear that invades many children and adults with an ID, which invades them like a default history? Mary (not her real name) had Down's syndrome and told me how difficult it was to go on a train or a bus. 'Everywhere I go, people look at me. I don't like them looking at me. I am not a film star. I have a disability. I can read and write a little. That is good. But people wish I was dead. Because my brain does not work the same as theirs. They are trying to stop babies with Down's syndrome being born.'

At the same time, a woman in a therapy group I co-convened, said: 'I know the worst word in the world.' The other women all nodded in agreement. It seemed they knew what this word was and could share it without saying it, even though they only met in the group and had no chance to talk privately. We asked the woman if she could say the word. She said she would need the group to help her. Syllable by syllable they uttered the word: 'Am'- 'ni'- 'o'- 'cen'- 'tes'-'is.' – 'amniocentesis' (Sinason, 2010).

The women did not disagree with abortion in general. Indeed, they said they might want an abortion if they knew they were carrying a disabled baby. It might be too hard for them to manage. But they hated the way film stars and celebrities said:

'I'm over 40, so I am having an amnio and if it is alright…'. They wanted women to say: 'Because I don't think I would be a good mother for a baby with a disability, sadly, I am having an amnio.'

Mary and the women in the group all came from loving families and in a country of peace. They had the rare resource of therapy. They had a voice. Through this, they could share the deepest fear that having an ID was a killing offence. There was a societal wish for them not to exist.

When I read of research to stop a baby eventually needing glasses, I feel excited. My identity is not linked to my glasses. But when you have an ID, it is part of your identity, your soul. How can you separate out someone stopping a new baby being born who has a disability, or repairing the disability in utero, from killing the child after it is born if you can actually feel the waves of murderousness around you?

The celebrated psychoanalytic historian Lloyd de Mause (1974) stated that childhood in most historical periods and even now in many countries was 'a nightmare from which we have only recently begun to awaken'. Sadly, the child or adult with an ID has similarly been traumatised in most periods of history with only glimmers of appropriate understanding and treatment. Disability has been, throughout the centuries, a hate crime that is allowed and which is acted upon.

De Mause saw the first stage of the history of childhood as infanticidal and I consider this holds true for disability history too. Only with disability, it did not just stop as a first stage of historical development. Ancient Roman and Greek laws allowed for the killing of weak or deformed children. This wish has not altered in most countries or in most periods of history. Indeed, even in countries that restrict a woman's rights over her own body, abortion is allowed at later stages if the foetus has a disability. Eugenics exists even when it is not named as such. Indeed, eugenics is a way of stopping the onward march of history, of stopping the possibility of people to have descendants. My late grandmother, who was a refugee with a mild ID through trauma, gave birth to a son who was to become the youngest medical professor of his time. She did not recognise letters but knew numbers. Each new degree he received she would put her tape measure across it to see how long the line of letters after his name had become! She loved him and was so proud of his learning. In a way, she was lucky that services did not exist when she was a young mother that would have removed her children from her.

Moments of light appear throughout history in the midst of the darkness and they deserve to be noted. Earlier, in the East, there was some concern for the handicapped. Confucius and Zoroaster, in the sixth century BC, instructed their followers to care for the 'weak-minded' and clothe them and treat them kindly.

A disciple of Confucius, Tzu-Chang explained in The Analects, written in about 500BC: 'I have heard that the gentleman honours his betters and is tolerant towards the multitude and that he is full of praise for the good while taking pity on the backward.'

However, it was a long period of hidden history before the reign of Constantine (312-337AD) in which the Bishop of Myra advocated protection of 'idiots' in monasteries (Penrose, 1963).

The role of religion, as we vividly know in our historical period, is mixed. On the one hand it offered a sense of protection when it considered all children and adults came under the care of the divine. But where there was a stronger concern about the 'satanic', fear and hatred could be projected to those who were different.

Looking over historical records we find the use of words that hurt us now but were considered kindly at the time. Reading through the next pages can cause hurt in reminding us of all the pain our citizens with an ID have experienced.

In 1198, Pope Innocent III initiated the monastic hospital tradition of humane care of the mentally ill and the disabled but, within the next 40 years, with religion as the strongest social force, any deviant behaviour was demonised. Families would throw out their own disabled members, scared they were devils, and those who received protection were a far smaller number. A Prussian law existed in 1230 that praised those who either left to die or burned the sick or feeble person.

 If people with a disability were spared the ordeals of the inquisition, they certainly faced a chilling 'death-making' (Wolfenburger, 1987) attitude of euthanasia. Against this, the small moments of good treatment stand out. In 1200AD, a church was erected in Gheel in honour of St Dymphna, who was born in 600AD and who fled an incestuous marriage with her father who pursued and killed her. She became a saint for those with mental maladies and children with ID were often left at the church which resulted in the beginnings of residential care of children with a disability (Khilgour, 1936).

During the reign of Edward I (1272-1307), there was a new legal concern about disability. In the Statute of Prerogatives, he defined the difference between born fools, 'fatuus naturalis', and 'unsound persons; who were 'non compos mentis'. While handicap among the poor was expected, any disability affecting the rich raised political problems. A born fool was not considered capable of change and, therefore, his property could be disposed of, whereas someone of unsound mind might recover. From Edward I to Edward VII at one level there was little change.

On 9 December 1484, Pope Innocent VIII issued a bill allowing more power to the Inquisitors. Disability, mental disease and sin were amalgamated, and death at the stake was the cruel medicine offered. Demonising, annihilation and only small pockets of concern can be seen. There is the frail beginning of institutional care via religion, as well as the concerns of framing the disabled as outside the care of religion and in the hands of the devil.

The Dark Ages did not end suddenly to make room for the Renaissance. There was a slow resurgence of the ancient Greek ideals and knowledge that Christianity had been unable to destroy. Aristotle was slowly allowed back, but demonic possession was still seen as the main cause of ID, impotence, phantom pregnancy and epilepsy.

The Protestant Luther (1576) believed the devil was the father of idiots and, on one occasion (Penrose, 1963), recommended a 12-year-old disabled child be drowned. He saw such children as changelings whose souls were taken over by the devil. Heinemann (2000) considers that while 'changelings', babies who were perceived as having been changed by faeries or demons, could be tolerated in medieval times, the view hardened in the 16th and 17th centuries. 'Although the children were still called "changelings" they were now considered to be the fruit of a sexual relationship between the devil and a witch.'

The 17th century added further torment for the mentally ill and those with intellectual disabilities. Descartes' famous dictum 'Cogito, ergo sum' meant that those who could not think were reduced to animal status, which, unlike in the East, meant being perceived as a dumb brute. The way to deal with a brute animal was to beat them into submission. Christian Franz Paullina wrote 'Flagellum Salutis' and believed that beatings were particularly useful for several diseases of the head including 'facial expressions of feeblemindedness' (Bromberg, 1954). As madness and disability became identified as animal unreason, the aggression of 'reasonable' society was liberated. Going to watch madmen and idiots perform behind bars enhanced the emotional distance made between the apparently thinking and non-thinking. Instead of being scared of the devil inside, the outside devil could be watched and tamed behind bars. This distancing made it possible to start building vast hospitals and asylums, what Foucault called 'the age of confinement'. Exclusion.

A 1655 decree in France declared workers holding guild meetings were guilty of sorcery. With unemployment and economic unrest, beggars were declared illegal and were the first to be confined. People who were poor, mentally ill or had an intellectual disability were moved from the streets and forced to work. Madness, disability and witchcraft were all linked.

In 1682, Louis XIV abolished the execution of witches and sorcerers and, in 1689, the English philosopher and father of Liberalism, John Locke differentiated between madmen and fools. The age of definitions and classifications was beginning. The religious demonising of the poor and disabled began to fade, but the care from monasteries was lost. Bethlehem Hospital moved from the religious umbrella to the hands of untrained overseers.

In England, the 1774 'Act for Regulating Madhouses' brought private mental hospitals under state regulation. The mental illness of George III fostered public interest in how to treat madness. This was the beginning of 'moral treatments'. In 1793, Philippe Pinel, who was against the use of physical force, was appointed physician of the Bicetre, which had 300 inmates. He freed people classified as lunatics and those with intellectually disability from their chains. His pupil, Jean-Etienne Dominique Esquirol, understood that 'idiocy is not a disease but a condition in which the intellectual faculties are never manifested'. Pinel and Esquirol established the foundations of psychotherapeutic psychiatry in France. In England, the Quaker, William Tuke, advanced the humane moral treatment and set up The Retreat at York, which was not a prison.

The end of the 18th century also saw the child-centred educational ideas of Rousseau inspire the teaching principles of the Swiss pioneer Pestalozzi (1746–1827), who devoted his life to teaching poor children. Rousseau and Pestalozzi both inspired Froebel (1782–1852), who encouraged the concept of free play. He saw children as plants that needed kindly interest.

In 1798, an adolescent was found in Aveyron who could not speak and behaved like an animal. Jean Itard, medical officer at the Institution for the Deaf and Dumb in Paris, applied his principles to the boy. Unlike Pinel, who felt the boy could never be educated, Itard was sure the absence of education and environment had handicapped the boy. Small improvements were made and this gave the idea that education might be of use.

Itard inspired Edouardd Seguin (1812–1880), a Christian socialist, who founded educational programmes at the Bicetre in 1842 and published a treatise, 'Idiocy: and its treatment by physiological method' (Seguin, 1866). Pope Pius IX welcomed Seguin's work, and by the end of the 19th century there were schools for the education of children with intellectual disabilities in America, Switzerland, Germany and England.

Seguin believed that individuals with an ID had been arrested at earlier stages of infancy or childhood. He emphasised that the disabled were part of humanity and that some aspects of handicap were curable. In 1837, he established the first school dedicated to the education of children with ID. He believed that an 'idiot' is endowed with a moral nature and is influenced by the same things as the rest of humanity (Seguin, 1846). However, there was still a link with animals, in that he stated that there is not one of any age who may not be made more of a man and less of a brute by patience and kindness directed by energy and skill (Seguin, 1846).

Each historical period continues with two lines of development, one in which there is progress in thinking and one in which the attacks on people with an ID continue. Interestingly, it is from this period that although people with ID and mental illness remained linked in the public mind, they had separate histories of provision.

In the UK, Andrew Reed in Highgate opened the first Asylum for Idiots with the patronage of Queen Victoria and the Prince Consort. At the same time in the USA, former schoolteacher Dorothea Dix started to give Sunday school lessons to women prisoners and she wrote to the United States Congress in 1848 on the appalling situation she witnessed: 'More than 9,000 idiots, epileptics and insane in the United States, destitute of appropriate care and attention, bound with galling chains, bowed beneath fetters and heavy iron balls attached to drag-chains, lacerated with ropes, scourged with rods and terrified beneath storms of execration and cruel blows; now subject to jibes and scorn and torturing tricks; now abandoned to the most outrageous violations.' She campaigned successfully for 40 years, causing major changes in the United States and England. (Sinason, 2003).

At the end of the 19th century, at the University of Pennsylvania, Lightner Witmer, who created the term 'clinical psychology', founded the first psychological clinic specifically for children with a handicap. He wanted to develop remedial methods as well as to understand why some 'normal' children were unable to use their intellectual skills. At the same time, American psychiatrist Walter Fernald founded the first scientific professional organisation to study handicap. In the United Kingdom, the 1886 Idiot's Act provided for the care of imbeciles and idiots. The 1899 Education Act distinguished between defective, epileptic and other children, and, in Italy, Dr Maria Montessori became interested in Seguin's work and pioneered educational ideas for children, including those with a disability.

Sadly, no moment of history that provided a step forward did not also reveal the opposite. In Germany, there was a 'growing stigmatisation of certain kinds of mental and physical handicap' (Evans, 2001), and compulsory certifications increased.

Evolutionary ideas then emerged through the writings of Lamarck (1744-1829) and then Darwin, who published the Origin of the Species in 1859. Francis Galton, Darwin's cousin, then created the term 'eugenics' and was convinced there was a 'curve of normal distribution', which meant there would always be a small group of exceptionally gifted and exceptionally handicapped people. Handicap was no longer ascribed to God in the same way as previously, but was seen as a blot on the landscape of man as a superior animal.

Eugenics had scientific blessing and was seen as modern. There was a realisation that while some changes could be made, a primary disability was immutable. There was now a new demonology of the poor and handicapped. The optimism that came from education was stopped. Genetics and eugenics were now the key words. In the United States, Witmer supported the 1911 Bill in the State of Pennsylvania to sterilise people with severe ID. Also in the US, Davenport (1911) advocated sterilisation and segregation of people with ID, and others wished to refuse any immigrant with a disability. Alfred Binet and James Cattell developed mental tests. Instead of murder there was eugenics. The age of the IQ had begun. The United States Congress passed the Immigration Act (1891) which barred 'lunatics, idiots, imbeciles and the feebleminded' from entering the USA. At Ellis Island in New York, 5,000 immigrants arrived each day. The immigration authorities put in place a screening process so that any arriving immigrant who presented with physical or mental difficulties was marked with a code in chalk on their clothes and sent for further assessment. Those screened and marked as having possible ID were then assessed on mental tests, such as the Seguin boards that are on display today at Ellis Island Museum. Those who failed the tests were refused admission and returned to their country of origin. Eighty-eight out of 100,000 immigrants were deported because they were deemed feeble-minded.

The impact of IQ tests was made more relevant by the beginning of the First World War and the issue of military recruitment. One-third of army recruits for the Boer War were considered intellectually unfit to serve. This provided devastating proof of cultural deprivation. When the first IQ tests revealed that most prostitutes and petty convicts were 'feeble-minded', even Walter Fernald (1859–1924), who cared about disability, supported sterilisation of intellectually disabled women. He was a man of his time in stating erroneous fearful comments such as: 'Feebleminded women are invariably immoral and if at large usually become carriers of VD or give birth to children who are as defective as themselves.' However, later in life he rejected forced sterilisations.

In 1908, the Radnor Commission in England found 'feeble-mindedness is largely inherited; that prevention of mentally defective persons from becoming parents would tend to diminish the number of such persons in the population'. The 1913 Mental Deficiency Act pursued the idea of segregation of the sexes and compulsory sterilisation continued up to the 1950s. Walmsley (2000) shows how 'women were targeted for sexual regulation and treated as mental defectives, depriving them of citizenship'.

From the 1920s, further classifications came that led equally to further provision and negatives. The improvements in societal attitudes and the persistence of irrational attitudes are almost equal.

The period leading to the Second World War marked a new step in eugenics. In Germany on 14 July 1933 the Law for the Prevention of Offspring with Hereditary Diseases demanded sterilisation for congenital "feeblemindedness" – what Hitler called 'domestic purification' in 1939. The original terminology of 'a merciful death' quickly changed to 'creatures unworthy of life' (Nazi circular, 1942).

The 1944 English Education Act changed the term "mental defective" to 'educationally subnormal' in the hope of creating a more humane attitude. The history of disability is filled with euphemisms whereby the term is changed in the hope of making a new period, only for that term to be seen as equally contaminating (Sinason, 2010).

In the past 50 years, within our own known history we see the familiar sights of more and more inclusive and thoughtful education Acts at the same time as lack of resources and awareness of higher-than-average abuse rates. In 1978, the Warnock report found 20% of children had special needs. I was very aware of this Act as my wonderful father, the late Professor SS Segal wrote his seminal book No Child is Ineducable to aid the passage of this Act. The 1981 Education Act brought in the term 'learning difficulties' and advocated normalising and inclusion. The 1989 Children Act, implemented in 1991, now accepted duty of care by local authorities for children who were not at school, and for all children in need in holidays and after school hours. Here, there was a new definition of 'children in need'. The 1993 Education Act defined special educational needs. The 2000 Carers and Disabled Children Act made provision for assessment of carers' needs and services to help carers, while the 2000 Committee on the Rights of the Child realised that abandonment and abuse were the consequences of stigma and institutionalisation. The 2001 Special Educational Needs and Disability Act made further provision against discrimination on the basis of disability. The 2014 Children and Families Act covered special educational needs and disabilities.

Where are we now? The best and the worst jostle alongside. The island of Leros housed children and adults with ID who were left tied up on their boards with no adequate food, education or medical care (Ramsay, 1990). In 2016, when 1,700 people in South Africa were moved from specialised care to unlicensed living, nearly 10% died. Residents were moved with no warning and without the knowledge of their families (Hodal and Hammond, 2018). Orphans in Romania were left without attachment figures to slowly deteriorate (Green, 2020). In 1995, China passed a eugenics law requiring prospective brides and grooms to have physical examinations (Mao, 1997). There are still parts of Japan where a mother who gives birth to a child with disability is expected to kill the baby and then herself to rule out the shame and dishonour to the family, and there is a remarkably non-retaliatory public response to such suicide-murders (Kawanishi, 1990). Sexual and physical abuse of children and adults with ID worldwide is widespread. The World Health Organization (Hughes *et al.*, 2012) states that both children and adults with disabilities are at much higher risk of physical and sexual violence than their non-disabled peers. Indeed, the United Nations Department of Economic and Social Affairs Fact Sheet on persons with disabilities (2021) reinforces this.

It is also important to note that, regardless of changes in the nature of religious belief and the growth of the concept of a loving deity, concepts of disability as sin or punishment never disappear.

Danquah (1976), looking at how children with severe intellectual disabilities were regarded in Ghana in the 1970s, found that educated and uneducated parents thought disability was linked to a curse from a supernatural being. Only 5% of educated, urban parents attributed the cause to genetic, biological or metabolic processes.

This history is a heavy one with only moments of light. May our friends, family and colleagues with an ID carry it as lightly as possible. The Institute for Psychotherapy and Disability was inaugurated in 2000 to ensure advocacy, enabling, rights for access to therapy, the innate right to be a sentient, sexual being. I hope this book shares the burden and allows a shift in the balance of the scales.

References

Bromberg P (1937, reprinted 1954) *The Mind of Man: A history of psychotherapy and psychoanalysis*. New York: Harper Torchbooks, Harper and Brothers.

Danquah SA (1976) A preliminary survey of beliefs about severely retarded children in Ghana. *Psychopathologie Africaine* **12** (2)1899-97.

Davenport C (1911) *Heredity in Relation to Eugenics*. New York: H. Holt and Company.

De Mause L (1974) *The History of Childhood*. London Souvenir Press.

Evans B, Wellcome Trust (2017) *The Metamorphosis of Autism. A history of child development in Britain*. Manchester University Press.

Evans, R (2001) Social outsider in German history (pp20-40). In: R Gellately (Ed) *Social Outsiders in Nazi Germany*. New Jersey, Princetown.

Green M F (2020) 30 years ago Romania deprived thousands of babies' human contact. The Atlantic, July/August.

Heinemann E (2000) *Witches, A Psychoanalytic Exploration of the Killing of Women*. Trans.

Hodal, K & Hammond R (2018). Emaciated, mutilated, dead: the mental health scadal that rocked South Africa. Guadian, 14th October 2018.

Kawanishi Y (1990) Japanese mother-child suicide; The psychological and sociological implications of the Kimura case. *Pacific Basin Law Journal* **8** (1) UCLA.

Jarrett S (2020) *Those they Called Idiots: The idea of the disabled mind from 1700 to the present day*. London: Reaktion Books.

Khilgour AJ (1936) Colonel Gheel. *American J of Psychiatry* **92** 959.

Mao, X (1997) Chinese eugenic legislation. *The Lancet*, **349** (9045) 139.

Penrose LS (1963) *The Biology of Mental Defect*. London: Sidgwick and Jackson.

Seguin E (1846) *Traitement Moral, Hygiene Et Education Des Idiots Et Des Autres Enfants Arrieres*. London: Bailliere Tindall.

Seguin, E (1866) *Idiocy: And its Treatment by Physiological Method*. New York: William Wood & Co.

Sinason V (2010) *Mental Handicap and the Human Condition: An analytic approach to intellectual disability*. London: Free Association Books.

Sinason V (2003) *Learning Disability as Trauma and the Impact of Trauma on Learning Disability*. PhD thesis, St George's Hospital Medical School, University of London.

Ramsay R (1990) Banished to a Greek island. *Psychiatric Bulletin*, **14**, 134-135.

United Nations Department of Economic and Social Affairs Fact Sheet on Persons with Disabilities, (undated) enable@un.org

Walmsley J (2000) Women and the Mental Deficiency Act of 1913: Citizenship, sexuality and regulation. *British Journal of Learning Disabilities* **28** (2) 65-70.

Wolfenburger W (1987) *The New Genocide of Handicapped and Afflicted People*. Syracuse: Syracuse University Division of Special Education and Rehabilitation.

Hughes K, Bellis M, Jones L, Wood S et al (2012) Prevalence and risk of violence against adults with disabilities; a systemic review and meta-analysis of observational studies *The Lancet*, **379** (9826) 1621-1629.

Chapter 4:
Freud, psychoanalysis, and trauma: significance in the acknowledgement and identification of trauma in the lives of people who have intellectual disabilities

Nigel Beail

Psychology, psychotherapy and psychiatry have a chequered history in relation to the acceptance of the relationship between trauma and psychological distress. In the 1980s the use of psychoanalytic psychotherapy started to be explored with people who have intellectual disabilities (ID). At the time Beail, Frankish and Sinason were among a small group of professionals pioneering this work. However, what is noticeable is that they identified that traumatic experiences were quite a common theme in the client's material, and this was reflected in their early case reports (Beail, 1989; Frankish, 1989; Sinason, 1988; 1992). Beail and Warden (1995) then published a paper from their psychodynamic psychotherapy clinic concerning 88 people with ID they had seen for therapy. They reported that 25% of the people they had seen disclosed sexual abuse during their therapy. Concurrent and subsequent research on the prevalence of sexual abuse of children and adults with ID then found similar figures (Horner-Johnson and Drum, 2006). This also was reflected in clinical reports (Sinason, 1999). At the same time there were the beginnings of paradigm shift in the understanding that trauma contributed to psychological distress (Ainscough and Toon, 1993; Mason, 1984). It is therefore not surprising that early, rather than contemporary, psychodynamic theories concerning the impact of trauma were turned to. When psychodynamic approaches began to be used with people who had ID in the 1980s, the prevalent view was the long-held position in the psychoanalytic world, as well as in other psychological theories, that trauma was largely caused by the patient's phantasies rather than real abuse; further when it was accepted the child reporting abuse was often called promiscuous. However, Freud's early work was more informed by reality as opposed to fantasy theory or blaming the individual, and it was to his early theories and those of his contemporaries that the pioneers in the provision of psychotherapy for people who have ID turned. In this chapter, these early trauma theories and their relevance will be outlined.

In 1896, Sigmund Freud presented a paper to his colleagues at the Society for Psychiatry and Neurology in Vienna on his discoveries working with his new method (Freud, 1896a), which he called psychoanalysis (Freud, 1896b). The seeds of Freud's ideas emerged in his book with Joseph Breuer, *Studies on Hysteria* (Freud and Breuer, 1893-1895). Both Beail (1989) and Sinason (1988; 1992) refer to Breuer and Freud's (1893-1895,) comment that 'the memory of trauma acts like a foreign body which long after entry must continue and be regarded as an agent still at work'. In 1896, in *The Aetiology of Hysteria*, Freud outlined an explicit theory that the origins of hysteria lay in early sexual traumas, drawing a link between traumatic experiences and psychological distress or psychiatric problems. The traumata Freud referred to in his paper included rape, abuse, and aggression. He described the psychoanalytic method as leading the patient's attention back from his presenting problem or symptom to the scene in which and through the symptom arose. Freud reported in his lecture that his analyses of 18 patients (six men and 12 women) had led to identifying a determinant of psychological distress that possesses the necessary traumatic force, and that these were sexual traumas in childhood. Freud reported that his patients had either experienced sexual assault at the hands of a stranger, or, more commonly, someone close to them such as a parent or care giver. He also reported discovering incestuous relationships in some cases. He put forward the theory that these distressing experiences were thrust out of conscious thought into the unconscious through the action of a defence he called repression. Freud also described how people presenting with psychological distress do so because a present-day precipitating event causes the past traumatic experiences to come into operation in the form of unconscious memories. It is the presence of these unconscious memories that give rise to the symptoms of psychological distress. Thus, a current traumatic or significant life event seems to bear no relation to the nature of the distress of the client as it links to the repressed, now unconscious trauma of the past. Freud put forward his new method of psychoanalysis to help the client on a path back to the memory of the earlier trauma. Basically, work on the recent trauma may not bring about psychological improvement as the recent trauma or event is unconsciously linked to an earlier, unresolved trauma. Freud found that behind the first traumatic scene there may be concealed the memory of a second or more scenes, whose reproduction has greater therapeutic effect. So, the first scene has the significance of a connecting link in the chain of associations to earlier scenes of greater traumatic force.

Freud also described a process identified in Beail (1989) and Sinason's (1992) case studies that came to be called 'acting out', whereby a child or adult feels compelled by their memory of sexual assault to repeat the same practices on another. Freud came to the view that sexual aggression in children was a result of their previous sexual assaultive experiences with an adult aggressor. Freud also speculated that sexual traumata had a causative role in a range of mental health difficulties. He stated that the aetiological role of childhood sexual experiences is not confined to hysteria, but holds good for obsessional problems and perhaps for various forms of chronic paranoia and other functional psychoses. Similarly, in the 1980s and 1990s clinicians were seeing abuse as a contributing factor to psychological distress in adults (Ainscough and Toon, 1993) and children, and adults who have ID (Beail and Warden, 1995; Turk and Brown, 1993; Vizard, 1989). Indeed, Beail and Warden (1995) concluded that 'acting out, sexualised play or behaviour, or other challenging behaviours may all be signs of sexual abuse' in people who have ID.

Freud did not stick to his theory and within the year he had shown clear signs of changing his mind. This period in Freud's life has been documented in detail by Mason (1984; 1992) and readers are referred to his book for a more in-depth account. According to Mason (1992), Freud's preoccupation with what was called his seduction theory ended abruptly in 1897 and this was communicated in a letter to his friend Wilhelm Fleiss, which is reproduced in Mason (1992). In the letter, Freud confided in his friend that he no longer believed in his trauma theory of hysteria. He explained that this was due to mixed results with his method, the surprise that it was fathers (not excluding his own) who were being perverse, and such widespread abuse against children are not very probable. However, Freud then wrote to Fleiss again, wavering and reporting another case where he accepted the client had been traumatised (Mason, 1992). In a paper in 1898, he again affirmed that sexual experiences in childhood are bound to be pathogenic (Freud, 1898). His first published reference to his abandonment of his trauma theory can be found in his book *Three essays on sexuality* (Freud, 1905), where he stated that he overrated the importance of seduction in comparison to other factors. In 1905, Freud explained that the material on which his trauma theory was based was scanty and happened by chance to include a disproportionately large number of cases in which sexual abuse by an adult or older child played a chief part of their childhood history. However, he does state that their accounts were not open to doubt, but that he overestimated the frequency of such events. In 1914, Freud wrote in *On the History of the Psychoanalytic Movement* that his 1896 paper was met with silence and thereafter he found himself in splendid isolation. He tried to understand his contemporaries' reactions through psychoanalytic theory. He stated that, 'if it was true that the set of facts I had discovered were kept from the knowledge of patients themselves by internal resistances of an affective kind, then these resistances would be bound to appear in healthy people too, as soon as some external source confronted them with what was repressed' (Freud, 1914; 1986a). Thus, for Freud the traumatic element in the sexual experiences of childhood lost its importance (Freud, 1953). The outcome was that he abandoned his theory in favour of the theory that his patients were having fantasies of, rather than experiences, of sexual assault and abuse.

Freud did not abandon his trauma theory completely. Mason (1992) states in a footnote that there is some evidence that, towards the end of his life, Freud (1940) once again was inclined to assign significance to sexual traumas in the genesis of neurosis, but the passages are too sketchy to permit definitive conclusion. Mason was referring to *An Outline of Psychoanalysis*, which Freud was unable to finish due to ill health and undergoing an operation. The manuscript was published posthumously in 1940 (Freud, 1940). In the chapter on 'an example of psychoanalytic work' Freud refers to things that may be described as a central experience in childhood. He goes on to say that our attention is first attracted to the effects of certain influences which do not apply to all children, though they are common enough – such as the sexual abuse of children by adults, older siblings or by seeing, at first hand, sexual behaviour between adults. Freud (1940) acknowledged that these occur at a time when a child would not be interested in or understand what was happening to them. However, he argued that such impressions would be subjected to repression either at once or as soon as they seek to return as memories and that they may result in neurosis, sexual perversion or sexual dysfunction. Thus, towards the end of his life, Freud was still accepting of trauma in his formulation of client's difficulties. However, he then said that a higher degree of interest must be attached to a situation all children go through, which flows from the prolonged period of being cared for and this is the Oedipus complex. Freud then explained his theories of children's sexual fantasies.

In addition to his 1940 mention of his trauma theory there are several other occasions when Freud refers to trauma, including childhood sexual assaults in his formulations of client difficulties. In his paper on the paths to the formation of symptoms (Freud, 1917), he summarised his position diagrammatically and traumatic experience is included. Later in the paper he explained that phantasies of being seduced are of particular interest, because so often they are not phantasies but real memories. However, he toned this down by adding that real memories do not occur as often as shown in his early work (Freud, 1896a) He did go on to warn that it would be wrong to suppose that sexual abuse of a child belongs entirely to the realm of phantasy. In terms of the outcome of psychoanalysis, Freud remarked that the outcome is the same whether phantasy or reality has the greater share in these events in childhood.

Beail (1989; 1994) and Sinason (1992) also described using the client's traumatic dreams in their clinical work. In *Beyond the pleasure principal* Freud (Freud, 1920) referred to different traumas such as accidents, war and incidents involving threats to life. Here he argued that dreams are the most trustworthy method of investigation. He observed that dreams occurring in those presenting with traumatic neuroses repeatedly take them back to the incident. He saw this as being fixated to the trauma. However, he also linked these traumas by quoting his earlier work where he stated that hysterics suffer from reminiscences (Freud and Breuer, 1895), which were, in those cases, sexual traumas. In *Beyond the Pleasure Principal* (Freud, 1920), Freud concluded that such an event as an external trauma is bound to provoke a disturbance on a large scale in the function of the organism's energy and to set in process every defensive measure. So, Freud was now seeing a range of traumatic experiences as having an impact on mental health. He took this up again in *Revision of dream-theory* (Freud, 1933) where he saw shock, severe psychical trauma (e.g. war) and childhood experiences of a traumatic nature as causes of traumatic hysteria.

In his last published case study of the wolf man, Freud (1918) referred to the man's observations of his parent having sex in his formulation; he then later commented that his attitude to female objects had been disturbed by an early seduction (Freud, 1926). However, the impact of the seduction is diminished as Freud saw the motive force being a fear of castration – the loss of his penis, the organ that distinguished him from a female. In his paper on female sexuality (Freud, 1931) he states that actual seduction is common enough and that it invariably disturbs the natural course of development and leaves behind extensive consequences. In *Moses and Monotheism* (Freud, 1938), Freud refers to a girl who was made the object of sexual seductions in early childhood and that this may direct her later sexual life so as to constantly provoke similar attention. Freud attributes to trauma a positive and negative function, and talks about analysis bringing the client to relive the trauma so a new sort of resolution of the trauma, more positive, more long-term, could take place.

Later, in an unfinished paper, Freud (1940b) described a boy who had become acquainted with the female genitals at a young age through being seduced by an older girl. However, Freud went on to discuss this in relation to castration anxiety as he did with the wolf man.

It seems that Freud also continued to waver in his views during his life. He struggled to understand presentations, such as those who are brought so completely to a stop by a traumatic event that shatters the foundation of his life and loses interest in the present and the future, and is absorbed by the past (Freud, 1917). In the main, Freud held to his fantasy theory, as did the whole psychoanalytic profession and those that developed from it, including psychiatry, psychotherapy and clinical psychology. However, Freud, over the years, seemed to continue to accept that real sexual trauma retains a certain aetiological importance (Freud, 1924), but a humbler one (Freud, 1925). He also referred to such events as 'no rare events' (Freud, 1926). It would seem that Freud lived with conflicting thoughts and feelings about his two theories, which he never completely resolved.

Freud's ideas soon became popular in many parts of the world and a psychoanalytic movement grew and institutes formed. The established view formed by the majority of the psychoanalysts was that of his fantasy theory and this held for nearly a century. Abraham (1907) purported a view that some children are precocious and show an abnormal desire for obtaining sexual pleasure, and that a sexual trauma is a masochistic expression of the sexual impulse. Freud's daughter, Anna, wrote to Mason in 1981 (Mason, 1992,) stating that keeping the seduction theory would mean abandoning the Oedipus complex, and with it the whole importance of conscious and unconscious phantasy life. In her view, there would have been no psychoanalysis without the abandonment of the seduction theory. However, this was not her father's view, as he saw fantasy and reality having the same impacts. But Anna Freud's view was shared by other analysts. For example, in his book, *The analytic experience*, published in the mid-1980s when psychodynamic work with people who have ID was just getting started, psychoanalyst Neville Symington states: 'When Freud gave up his theory that neuroses were triggered by the seduction of a patient by her father or another close male relative, he came to the truth that phantasied wishes were the source of mental disturbance' (Symington, 1986. Symington is credited with the publication of the first case study of working psychoanalytically with a person with ID (Symington, 1981), but he did not continue to do so (Sinason, 1992; 1999).

Notable exceptions in Freud's lifetime were Sandor Ferenczi and Melanie Klein. In 1932 Ferenczi presented a paper about the impact of the reality of sexual abuse on children. Interestingly, when Ferenczi presented his paper expressing these views before the 12th International Psycho-Analytic Congress he, like Freud before him, met with disapproval (Masson, 1992). In his paper, Ferenczi (1932) returns to Freud's 1896 theory and argued as Freud did before him based on his analytic work, that trauma, specifically sexual trauma, cannot be stressed enough as a pathogenic agent. He also argued that the idea we are dealing with sexual fantasies of the child or hysterical lies is weakened by the multitude of confessions to sexual assaults on children by patients in analysis. In addition to sexual assaults, Ferenczi also talked about unbearable punishments and enraged punitive sanctions, and their depressive consequences for the child. Whereas Freud (1896a) largely focused on the abused child's effort to repress the memory into the unconscious, Ferenczi described their impact as causing a range of psychological reactions, including the defences of splitting of the personality, regression, fixation, fragmentation, identification with, and introjection of the aggressor. He also described the emergence of behaviours that are challenging, pathogenic progression and precocity, and depression. He additionally observed in his patients that the trauma they experienced can give rise to horrific fantasies derived from the real event. Ferenczi concluded that if all of what he states is true we shall be obliged to revise certain chapters of psychoanalytic theory. He advised analysts to pay closer attention to the strange, much veiled, yet critical manner of thinking and speaking of your children, patients and students, and so to speak, loosen their tongues; you will hear much that is instructive. Ferenczi's paper did not fit with the accepted theory of psychoanalysis at the time. According to Mason (1984), the reaction was uniformly negative. The paper was published in 1932 in German but not in English. It was translated into English by Ernest Jones, but Ferenczi died in May 1933, and Jones pulled its publication. It was later translated into English again and published in 1949, and again in 1984 (Mason, 1992). Thus, by the time Ferenczi presented his paper, between him and Freud, the impact of trauma on a child and later the adult were clear, but not accepted, but concur with the clinical observations of Finkelhor (1986): traumatic sexualisation, stigmatisation, betrayal and powerlessness.

Melanie Klein began psychoanalysis with Ferenczi in 1914. She then became a pupil of Ferenczi's, and with his encouragement, developed child analysis. Following the upheaval of the First World War and the new political situation in Hungary, Klein moved to Slovakia and then in 1921 to Berlin. In Berlin she made links with the founder of the German Psychoanalytical Society and clinic, Karl Abraham, and began providing child analysis at the clinic. According to Klein's biographer, Grosskurth (1986), it is the children she analysed in Berlin that are those in her book *The Psychoanalysis of Children* (Klein, 1932). Abraham became her analyst at the beginning of 1924, but this came to an end when he fell ill in the summer of 1925. Abraham had a very different view to Ferenczi and subscribed to Freud's fantasy theory. Freud also referred to Abraham's view that some children show an abnormal desire for obtaining sexual pleasure, and because of this undergo sexual trauma (Abraham, 1907). In Berlin, Klein was developing her play technique but was received with increasing ostracism and abuse from those close to Freud. Not that she was seen as aligning herself with the trauma model, but because she was developing ideas contrary to those of others developing child analysis in Vienna. She was invited to present a series of lectures in London in 1925, which were well received, and then was invited to move there, which she did in 1926.

Klein missed the Wiesbaden Congress of 1932 and so missed Ferenczi's controversial presentation on sexual abuse and trauma. However, Klein must have had some familiarity with Ferenczi's thesis as she had known him since 1914. Indeed, Grosskurth (1986) argues that Ferenczi had a lasting impact on her thinking and we can see in her work the elements she took from him and developed notably his use of active technique in her development of play technique, attention to the negative transference, omnipotence, introjection and using symbols. However, in a foot note Grossgurth (1986), argues that if Klein had attended the 1932 Congress it would have caused a confrontation, since what Ferenczi said was contrary to all that she believed. However, her accounts of psychoanalytic work in The Psychoanalysis of Children (Klein, 1932) would tend to contradict this or show that she had some acceptance of the impact of real traumatic events in her formulations. Klein describes the analyses of several children in the book and in several accounts, she reports on sexual activities and abuse in childhood.

In analysis of a child called Fritz (Klein, 1925) who presented with tics, Klein reported several traumatic experiences in his history. He had his foreskin stretched at the age of three, and until the age of six occupied a cot in his parents' bedroom, exposed to their sexual activities. The boy was also beaten by his father for cowardice and if caught masturbating.

In Klein's accounts of the analysis of Rita, Erna and Peter (Klein, 1932), her formulations also took into account the impact of having all witnessed their parents' sexual relations. In her formulation in the case of Peter she states that in his first analytic session he demonstrated the connection between the banging together and destruction of his toys with his observations of coitus. Peter's behaviour here would be described as acting in the transference. Peter is then reported to be acting out sexually with his brother and that his sexual relations with his brother were based on an identification with his father and mother. Klein's approach was to see the child's play in the same way as the adults' free associations. She therefore interpreted the child's repetitive behaviour of banging toys together as the parents banging their genitals together, which she linked to the child's observation of their parents having sex. Klein refers to Peter again in her later work on play technique (Klein, 1955), where she again makes the link in her formulation between the change in Peter's mental health, or as she put it 'a great impact on his mind' (Klein, 1955) and the witnessing of his parents having sex.

When Klein introduces the case of Kenneth (Klein, 1932) she states that he was seduced by his nurse. However, the boy was conscious of the event. Kenneth had been taken into the bath with his nurse where he had to rub her genitals. Kenneth did not report anything negative about the nurse, but did report recurring dreams of touching an unknown woman's genitals and masturbating her. Klein reported that in his analysis she found that he was in fear of his nurse. However, Klein then introduces elements of phantasy theory, for she states Kenneth linked the fear of his nurse to the fear of his bad mother and castrating father. In Kenneth's dream, the castrating father is represented by a man shooting his ear off in the bathroom – the place where he had masturbated his nurse. However, what this shows is that Klein was incorporating the real trauma of sexual abuse into her formulation, much in the way Freud did in his 1896 paper and later with the wolf man and the boy in his 1940b paper.

In the case of Ludwig, Klein (1932) referred to sexual relations with his younger brother and that the boy forced his younger brother into them. She reported Bill (aged 15 years) recalled some sexual acts with another boy, and Mr B, a man in his mid-thirties, being abused by his brothers in childhood. In the analysis of brothers Gunther and Franz she reported tracing back to mutual sexual acts. Here the elder brother, Gunter, forced his younger brother to perform fellatio, masturbation and anal touching. In one session, Klein described Franz threatening her with a wooden spoon and wanting to push it in her mouth, calling her small, stupid and weak. Klein stated: 'The spoon symbolised his brother's penis being forcibly thrust into his own mouth.' Klein reported that the boy had acted this out with other children and turned the hatred against himself and to her in the transference situation. It is clear from reading this that Klein was of the view that Franz had been sexually abused and that his communications in the therapy session were that of abuse and not of some unconscious phantasy of being abused by his brother. Indeed, she expressed concerns as to what we now call safeguarding.

There are also two footnotes in *The Psychoanalysis of Children* about incest and child abuse. In one, Klein noted that sexual relations between children are more frequent even during latency and puberty than is usually supposed. Then in another footnote on the impact of abuse she stated that this is more the case where a child has been seduced or raped by an adult. Klein stated that such an experience, as is well known, can have very serious effects upon a child's mind.

Unfortunately, Klein's (1955) later works have few references to the impact of trauma and abuse. Further, writings on her work seem to have avoided references to trauma and child abuse. For example, Hinshelwood (1994) referred to Klein's analysis of Peter and described Peter's play but avoided any reference to Peter's observation of his parent having sex in her formulation, and instead saw Klein as helping Peter put his fantasy into words. *The Dictionary of Kleinian Thought* (Hinshelwood, 1991) and *The New Dictionary of Kleinian Thought* (Bott Spillius, Milton, Garvey, Couve and Steiner, 2001) make no reference to trauma in their discussion of child analysis, even though they refer to Klein's formulations of her work with Felix, Rita, Erna and Peter. Klein's successors, like Freud's, have stayed loyal to the role of phantasy to the exclusion of reality in their work. However, Klein (1932) shared Freud's view that the 'causation of neuroses are complex and cannot be influenced in general if we take account of only a single factor' (Freud, 1918 quoted in Klein, 1997).

In 1914, when Freud was reflecting on the reaction to his 1886 theory, he asked how he could compel healthy people to examine it in a cool and scientifically objective spirit. He concluded this was best left to time to clear up. However, he went on to say that in the history of science, one can see that often the proposition that has called out nothing but contradiction, has later been accepted. But at the time, Freud concluded that no new proofs in support of it have been brought forward. However, he did not seem to have fully given up on his theory and was still affirming the role of psychoanalysis in the treatment of people who have experienced real traumas. He argued that the correct reconstruction of such forgotten experiences always has a great therapeutic effect, whether they permit objective confirmation or not (Freud, 1926b).

In their work with adults and children who have ID from the mid-1980s, Beail (1989); Beail and Warden, (1995); Frankish, (1989); and Sinason (1992) were reporting similar findings to Freud (1896a), Ferenzci (1932) and Klein, (1932), and continued to do so (Beail and Newman, 2005; Sinason, 2000), along with others providing psychodynamic psychotherapy (see, for example, Cottis, 2009). However, they approached psychoanalytic or psychodynamic psychotherapy with fresh eyes, with a population who had been viewed as unsuitable recipients. This was also a time when opinion was changing and sexual abuse was being recognised as an issue that needed to be addressed in society, and that victims needed to be believed and helped therapeutically (Ainscough and Toon, 1987). In case studies – for example, Ali (Sinason, 1992) and Alan (Beail and Newman, 2005), clients are observed to act sexually in the session with and towards the therapist. This was accepted as communication in the transference relationship of real traumatic events in the same way Klein (1932) understood and accepted what became called the "acting in" communications in the transference from Peter and Franz. The emerging literature on psychoanalysis, psychoanalytic and psychodynamic psychotherapy with people who have ID (Beail and Jackson, 2013; Frankish, 2016; Jackson and Beail, 2013; Sinason 2010) has developed in line with a more contemporary psychoanalytic view grounded in Freud's pre-1897 theory. Additionally, they have embraced the work of child analysts and psychotherapists and the understanding of emotional development, and earlier means of defence against trauma.

References

Abraham K (1907) The experiencing sexual trauma as a form of sexual activity. In: *Selected Papers of Karl Abraham* (1973) (pp47–63). London: Hogarth.

Ainscough C & Toon K (1993) *Breaking Free: Helping survivors of child sexual abuse*. London: Sheldon Press

Beail N (1989) Understanding Emotions: The Kleinian approach explained. In: D Brandon (Ed) *Mutual Respect: Therapeutic approaches to working with people with learning difficulties* (Ch.3, pp27–43). Surrey, Good Impression.

Beail N (1994) Fire, coffins and skeletons In: V Sinason (Ed) *Treating Survivors of Satanist Abuse*. London: Routledge.

Beail, N, & Jackson, T (2013). Psychodynamic psychotherapy. In: JL Taylor, WR Lindsay, R Hastings and C.Hatton (Eds) *Psychological Therapies for People with Intellectual Disabilities* (pp237–252). Chichester: Wiley.

Beail N & Newman D (2005) Psychodynamic counselling and psychotherapy for mood disorders. In: P Sturmey (Ed) *Mood Disorders in People with Mental Retardation*. New York: NADD Press.

Beail N &Warden S (1995) Sexual abuse of adults with learning disabilities. Journal of Intellectual Disability Research 39 (5) 382–387.

Bott-Spillius E, Milton J, Garvey P, Couve C & Steiner D (2011) *The New Dictionary of Kleinian Thought*. London: Routledge.

Breuer J & Freud S (1893-1895) *Studies in Hysteria. The standard edition of the complete psychological works of Sigmund Freud. Vol. 2*. London: Hogarth

Cottis T (Ed) (2009) Intellectual Disability, Trauma and Psychotherapy. London: Routledge

Ferenzci S (1932) Confusion of tongues between adults and the child. Translation by J Masson and M Loring In J Masson (1992) *The Assault on Truth: Freud and Child Sexual Abuse* (pp291–303). London: Fontana.

Finkelhor D (1986) *A Source Book in Child Sexual Abuse*. London: Sage.

Frankish, P (1989). Meeting the emotional needs of handicapped people: a psychodynamic approach. *Journal of Mental Deficiency research* 33: 407–14.

Frankish P (2016) *Disability Psychotherapy: An innovative approach to trauma-informed care*. London: Karnac.

Freud S (1896a) The Aetiology of Hysteria. *The standard edition of the complete psychological works of Sigmund Freud. Vol. 3* (pp191–221). London: Hogarth.

Freud S (1896b) Further Remarks on the Neuro-psychoses of Defence. *The standard edition of the complete psychological works of Sigmund Freud. Vol. 3*. London: Hogarth.

Freud S (1898) Sexuality and the Aetiology of the Neuroses. *The standard edition of the complete psychological works of Sigmund Freud. Vol. 3*. London: Hogarth.

Freud S (1905a) Three Essays on the Theory of Sexuality. *The standard edition of the complete psychological works of Sigmund Freud. Vol. 7*. London: Hogarth.

Freud S (1906) My Views on the Part Played by Sexuality in the Aetiology of the Neuroses. *The standard edition of the complete psychological works of Sigmund Freud. Vol. 7* (pp270–279). London: Hogarth.

Freud S (1914) On the History of the Psychoanalytic Movement. *The standard edition of the complete psychological works of Sigmund Freud. Vol. 14*. London: Hogarth.

Freud S (1917) The Paths to the Formation of Symptoms. Lecture 23 In Introductory Lectures on Psychoanalysis. *The standard edition of the complete psychological works of Sigmund Freud. Vols 15-16.* London: Hogarth.

Freud S (1918) From the History of Infantile Neurosis. *The standard edition of the complete psychological works of Sigmund Freud. Vol. 17.* London: Hogarth.

Freud S (1920) Beyond the Pleasure Principle. *The standard edition of the complete psychological works of Sigmund Freud. Vol. 18.* London: Hogarth.

Freud S (1924) Footnote added to Freud, 1896b The Neuro-psychoses of Defence. *The standard edition of the complete psychological works of Sigmund Freud. Vol. 3* (pp 221–243). London: Hogarth.

Freud S (1925) Autobiographical Study. *The standard edition of the complete psychological works of Sigmund Freud. Vol. 20* (pp 33–34). London: Hogarth.

Freud S (1926b) The Question of Lay Analysis. *The standard edition of the complete psychological works of Sigmund Freud. Vol. 19.* London: Hogarth

Freud S (1926a) Inhibitions, Symptoms and Anxiety. *The standard edition of the complete psychological works of Sigmund Freud. Vol. 20.* London: Hogarth.

Freud S (1931) Female Sexuality. *The standard edition of the complete psychological works of Sigmund Freud. Vol. 21* (pp 221-43). London: Hogarth.

Freud S (1933) Revision of Dream Theory. Lecture 29 In New Introductory Lectures on Psychoanalysis. *The standard edition of the complete psychological works of Sigmund Freud. Vol. 22.* London: Hogarth.

Freud S (1938) Moses and Monotheism. *The standard edition of the complete psychological works of Sigmund Freud. Vol. 23.* London: Hogarth.

Freud S (1940a) An Outline of Psychanalysis. *The standard edition of the complete psychological works of Sigmund Freud. Vol. 23.* London: Hogarth.

Freud S (1940b) Splitting of the Ego in the Process of Defence. *The standard edition of the complete psychological works of Sigmund Freud. Vol. 23.* London: Hogarth.

Grosskurth P (1986) *Melanie Klein: Her world and her work.* London: Aronson.

Hinshelwood RD (1991) *A Dictionary of Kleinian Thought* (2nd Ed). London: Free Association.

Hinshelwood RD (1994) *Clinical Klein.* London: Free Association

Hollins, S & Sinason V (2000). New perspectives: Psychotherapy, learning disabilities and trauma. *British Journal of Psychiatry* **176**, 32–36.

Horner-Johnson W & Drum CE (2006) Prevalence of maltreatment of people with intellectual disabilities: a review of recently published research. *Mental Retardation and Developmental Disabilities Research Review* **12**, 57-69.

Jackson T, & Beail N (2013). The practice of individual psychodynamic psychotherapy with people who have intellectual disabilities. *Psychoanalytic Psychotherapy* **27**, 108–123.

Klein M (1925) A contribution to the psychogenesis of tics. *International Z Psychoanal* **11** 332–349.

Klein M (1932) *The Psychoanalysis of Children.* London: Hogarth.

Klein M (1955) *Envy and Gratitude.* London: Hogarth.

Mason J (1984) *The Assault on Truth: Freud and Child Sexual Abuse.* New York: Farrar, Strauss & Giroux Inc.

Mason J (1992) *The Assault on Truth: Freud and child sexual abuse.* London: Fontana.

Mollon P (2000) *Freud and False Memory Syndrome.* Cambridge: Icon Books.

Sinason V (1988) Smiling, swallowing, sickening and stupefying: the effect of abuse on the child. *Psychoanalytic Psychotherapy* **4** 97–111.

Sinason V (1992) *Mental Handicap and the Human Condition: New approaches from the Tavistock.* London: Free Association Books.

Sinason V (1999) Psychoanalysis and Mental Handicap: Experience from the Tavistock Clinic. In: J De Groef & E Heinemann (Eds) *Psychoanalysis and Mental Handicap.* London: Free Association.

Sinason V (2010) *Mental Handicap and the Human Condition: An analytic approach to intellectual disability.* London: Free Association.

Symington N (1981) The psychotherapy of a subnormal patient. *British Journal of Medical Psychology* **54** 187–199.

Symington N (1986) *The Analytic Experience: Lectures from the Tavistock.* London: Free Association Books.

Turk V & Brown H (1993) Sexual abuse of adults with learning disabilities: results of a two-year incidence survey. *Mental Handicap Research* **6** 193–216.

Vizard E (1989) Child sexual abuse and mental handicap: a child psychiatrist's perspective. In: H Brown & A Craft (Eds) *Thinking the Unthinkable* (pp18–27). London: FPA.

Chapter 5:
Early development affected by early trauma

Pat Frankish

This chapter, based on over 30 years of experience, of working with people of all ages and all levels of disability, has led me to an understanding of the impact of early trauma on the development of the self, personality, and whole identity. This work has been demanding, emotional, productive, and has led me to a position of wanting to share what I have found with my colleagues and, more importantly, people who are affected by trauma.

The work is based primarily on that of Margaret Mahler and her colleagues, who were working in the 1970s in the USA. In her book, *The Psychological Birth of the Human Infant*, written with her colleagues Pine and Bergman, Mahler describes a stage process of emotional development (Mahler, Pine and Bergman, 1975). Traditionally, early development is measured in physical development and cognitive development, with less attention paid to indications of successful emotional development. It is difficult to know whether that is because it is too difficult or because it is too painful to accept that little children have the experiences of trauma that affect their whole development. My own work, which is labelled primarily TIC, also includes reference to the work of Donald Winnicott, John Bowlby, Melanie Klein, Wilfred Bion and Sigmund Freud (Frankish, 2016). Freud tended to veer away from looking at early child development, but he was the father of psychoanalysis, and the first person to publish work about the emotional world of people and the impact of early-life experiences on the adult self. The other writers I mention all spoke and wrote extensively about early development and the impact of failures in the process. What I hope to do within this chapter is to summarise the work, the usefulness of the model, and provide some examples of its use that have been quite dramatic in their impact.

So how did I get started in this work? I grew up in the grounds of a long-stay hospital where my parents worked. I was familiar, from a very young age, with people with disabilities and a range of behaviour that I didn't begin to understand. But I accepted that the people were people because that was the way I was brought up. At a later stage, in my early twenties, I went to work in that same hospital. I had three children myself by this stage and I worked school hours only as a play leader on what was then called a back ward, with 16 women who were too disturbed or distressed to go out to the occupational therapy department, or the other activities that were available. At the time, a trainee psychologist was allocated to the hospital for six months, and she saw in me somebody who could work with her and carry on with her ideas on the days that she was not there. From her, I learned about the differences between attention seeking and affection seeking, the impact of cognitive impairment on the ability to interact with the world, and the impact of the environment on behaviours that were seen as antisocial or certainly unsocial. I had no formal training at that stage, but had a brain, and I had to work out how to help the 16 women. All 16 together were certainly overwhelming. The first thing I did was to carry out some very preliminary assessments. These included a nine-piece jigsaw, a screwing and unscrewing rod, a stacking toy, and pencil and paper. It is important to bear in mind that the 16 women were considered to be severely intellectually disabled and not able to function at anything like an ordinary level. In carrying out my initial assessments, I discovered that several of them had more ability of a cognitive nature than was assumed. From those initial assessments I separated them into four groups of four and then provided activities in a small, separate room for each group. They had an hour a day and each group got one session a day. I discovered very quickly that they responded positively to more individual attention and had abilities that had not been recognised before. It also became clear that some of them had quite serious emotional pain. I think I may have been aware of that, more so than their nursing staff, because I had no responsibility for their physical well-being or the maintenance of the environment.

It became obvious quite quickly that the environment of living in a restricted space with 40 people when everybody was in, and certainly 40 people at mealtimes, was stressful. The ability to be an individual in that environment is extremely difficult and it became clear that certain behaviours were linked to identity. So, one woman would become known as the one who stole food, and another would be known as the one who always wet herself at mealtimes, and so on. It was almost as though that was the only way to be an individual. It was as if the behaviour became the person and that is something that I have noticed again and again, and still do, to this day. It is not quite as bad as it was back in the 1960s and 1970s when people were described by their behaviours, but it can still be an issue in schools and in residential settings for people to be described as the one who steals, the one who shouts, the one who scratches, or the one who screams. The ability to claim an identity has changed over the years, but still has some way to go.

Having met the psychology trainee during this job, and with her encouragement, I set out to become qualified as a clinical psychologist. As you can imagine, this took many years. When I qualified, I had to consider which specialty area I would choose to practice in. During my training, I was very taken by adult psychotherapy, by forensic work, and by child work. But my early experience of living and working with people with intellectual disabilities gave me skills for communicating and interacting that it seemed a shame to waste. So, I took the option to follow my career in that specialty. But, as I had not lost my interest in other areas of psychology, I have, throughout my career, maintained a generic caseload. Initially, I did this by seeing parents and siblings for therapy and, initially, services for people who have intellectual disabilities were cradle to grave, so there was lots of opportunity to work with all age groups. When the government decided that children were children first and so their services were to be provided by children's services, I opted to work in adult services but started a small, private practice to ensure that I could keep a generic caseload. In adult services, in various roles I took on management responsibility and forensic opportunities. What this has enabled me to do is to test out my growing interest in the link between early-life experiences, trauma and identity.

In my first qualified role, I was a member of a psychotherapy supervision group in Yorkshire of clinicians who were pioneering the provision of psychotherapy to people who have intellectual disabilities. It was in that group that I was first introduced to the work of Margaret Mahler. I bought her book and was struck immediately by the similarity between her description of the behaviours that she saw in young children, and the behaviours that I saw in the adults with intellectual disability (ID) who were very distressed or disturbed. Then the authority that I was working for had taken on responsibility for closing the hospital where I had worked many years previously. This meant that I was working with the same people, whose behaviours had not changed in 20 to 30 years, and looking to their future. At the same time, I was being referred children who were showing signs of distress, most of whom were in receipt of respite care because the families were struggling to support them. Some of these children were fostered or adopted because their family of origin either could not manage or were not able to provide adequate care. I worked with a number of children and adults using the model from Mahler and that work was published, initially presented at the International Association for the Scientific Study of Intellectual and Developmental Disabilities Congress in Dublin in 1988 and published in 1989 (Frankish, 1989).

So, what does the book say? What Mahler and her colleagues did was to establish a human laboratory where they studied the behaviour of children with their significant other, usually their mother, from nought to five years of age. In the sessions in the laboratory, the observers were able to chart the development of behaviour through time, and to notice if the progression was not smooth. Together with the identifiable features that may or may not influence the smooth progression, they noticed if the relationship between mother and child, child and mother, was relaxed or strained, cold or warm, positive or negative. From those observations, they were able to identify specific observable behaviours that were associated with different stages of development. This included a progression that was common to all the children, so took on the features of something that was developmentally specific to the development of human children. So, the period that was charted was from biological birth; the time at which the child arrives in the world, and psychological birth; the point at which the child can be separate from its primary carer and have manageable anxiety. At no point is there an assumption that there will be no anxiety because some anxiety is necessary for survival. If human beings had no anxiety, they would put themselves at risk and would potentially die, so some anxiety is healthy.

We come to a description of the stages, which I know I have done elsewhere, but this chapter would not be complete without the reference point. The first stage Mahler described as the symbiotic stage. This is the stage after birth and for a few weeks where mother and child are so close that it is as if they are still joined together. It was noted that some dyads of mother and child were more relaxed with the symbiotic stage than others. It was also noted that some mothers and babies must be separated at this critical time because one or the other is ill and needs further medical attention. If all goes well, the symbiotic stage is progressed positively, mother and baby are relaxed with each other, in tune with each other, and move on to the next stage.

The next stage is called differentiation. This was noted by the observers as the point at which the baby begins to take notice of its immediate surroundings and its own body. The child begins to play with its toes, look at its fingers, and play with the sides of the cot or the toys across the front of the pram. They are differentiating between themselves and their immediate surroundings. I mention here, because it may be useful, that this stage is also seen in advanced dementia, when people have lost much of their ability and their world becomes the chair or their bed and what they notice is what is in their immediate surroundings or their own body. The baby in the differentiation stage will respond with a smile but does not make any distinction about who they will smile for.

After a few months of the differentiation stage, the baby becomes able to do things. The first thing that they become able to do usually is roll over. When they can rollover, they do so again and again and again. This is described as practising. The child will practise the new skill that has become available to them, until proficient, and then that skill is filed away in the repertoire of behaviours, and a new skill is practised. So, rolling over is fun until you can sit up, sitting up is fun until you can crawl and crawling is fun until you can walk. In between, you learn to throw things, to grab things, to pull your mother's hair, and so on. This practising behaviour is more common, frequent and complex if there is feedback from the primary carer. What is particularly noticeable is that the child in the practising stage does not initiate interaction with the adult. The behaviour is totally self-generated and for self-satisfaction. This is a really important point to note, particularly for adults with intellectual disabilities (or not), as the behaviour can be described as obsessive, repetitive, or autistic. As part of ordinary development, it is part of the process of the child experimenting with its own skill development. If it becomes stuck at the practising stage for some reason, then the behaviours will be retained and will look autistic. It becomes a question of diagnosis when looking at the difference between autism and trauma-induced restriction in the development of the emotional self. The stage of practising generally lasts for a few months around the age of one so perhaps from ten to 14 or 15 months. The shift to the next stage is often linked to the ability to walk and to speak.

Once a child can walk and speak, it is able to run away, and to say no. This is the point at which interaction begins, and the child begins to initiate contact. It moves from being a recipient of attention and interest and support, to being much more demanding and choosing what it wants and what interests. In ordinary neuro-typical development, the beginning of this stage, called early rapprochement, is exciting and fun, and most parents enjoy it. However, if it persists for years and years it tends to become labelled as attention-seeking behaviour. This is the sort of labelling that I would have found in my early work with people with intellectual disabilities. The people labelled as attention seeking were given less attention, which is completely illogical. This stems from a belief that the attention was wanted rather than needed. This model of understanding emotional development makes it very clear that the behaviour means attention is needed, not just wanted. So, early rapprochement, the beginnings of two-way interaction, is a crucial stage in the development of the self in relation to other people – in other words, the social being that human beings are. Interruption of this process at this stage is critical in terms of the ability to function well as an adult. Children, with or without disabilities, who have experienced trauma at this stage (about 15-to-24 months) will suffer some sort of consequence. Trauma is idiosyncratic: the child will react to what it reacts to, and no two children are the same. It is possible to identify when a child has been traumatised because their development slows down and stops. It can be assumed that the development has stopped because of some brain development issue or illness that has been missed. What is rarely acknowledged is that the child has been traumatised by something that seemed like a perfectly ordinary event to the adults around them. Sadly, one of the common traumatic events is the arrival of a sibling. The arrival of a new baby changes the whole world for the toddler who suddenly is meant to be grown up, and may even be expected to help to look after this very noisy bundle that needs so much attention.

Early rapprochement moves on to late rapprochement and this involves the gradual development of negotiation and meaningful two-way interaction. The two-way interaction that began with early rapprochement involved mostly games, turn taking and the beginnings of recognition that two-way interaction has meaning, and that the other person may have views of their own. In the late rapprochement stage, there is gradually more recognition and acceptance of the fact that, in the two-way interaction, both parties have a role and rights and responsibilities. The process continues with a gradual increase in negotiation and decision-making that is shared, and the maturation of the child, to a point at which they have a clear separate identity and personality from the parent. In *The Psychological Birth of The Human Infant* (1975) Mahler described something that she called the rapprochement crisis, the point at which the child can be separate with manageable anxiety. If you are observing a room full of three- to four-year-olds, you will see that some of them are checking in with adults at regular intervals and some of them are not. The ones who are have not quite reached the crisis yet, and the ones who aren't already have. Or, sadly, they have given up on adults as being there for them. The latter group are the ones who will have more difficulty as their life progresses. There can be no doubt that in a room full of adults there will be some who have not fully progressed to having a secure psychological identity. In Balint terms, these would be described as those with a basic fault, with an ontological psychological wound that has become a scar and will not therefore heal, but can be adapted to and lived with (Balint, 1979).

The simplicity of this model and the ease with which the stage can be identified, has, to me, become what I see as its value. There are reams and reams of books and texts and research studies of mental health issues, and of behaviour problems in children and adults with disabilities that look for descriptions, meanings and interventions. Many of them seem to have a complicated and very wordy explanation for behaviour. It is my contention that this simple model can explain so much, if we accept that little children can be traumatised by what would seem to be ordinary events. Of course, some children are traumatised by horrendous events, but they are more readily recognised. The measurement tool became my doctoral study and has been further developed and published in 2019 (Frankish, 2019).

I want to go on now to talk about how the other clinicians I have mentioned contribute to my understanding of this way of seeing the development of self.

Donald Winnicott, John Bowlby, and Melanie Klein were all working at approximately the same time, all living in London, and all very much in tune with each other. They were all committed to early experience for children and the impact that had on their adult self. Freud had indicated that children were not seriously engaged in their long-term development until the age of seven. These three people challenged that and there is now very much support for their position. The key factors each have to contribute to what I am saying here will be enlarged on now.

Winnicott was a prolific writer, and there is much literature worthy of reading. I will limit myself here to his first seminal work *The Child the Family and the Outside World*, which talks about early development of the child within the family and then how they join the outside world (Winnicott, 1964). He stresses the need for a strong bond between mother and child and emphasises that the biological relationship is the best one, but others can be a substitute – they will just be different. He talks about the way the mother keeps the child in mind, and how that helps the child to develop with manageable anxiety. He goes on to describe the way the child has a one-person relationship with itself and as a new baby is very much not connected emotionally. That quickly becomes a two-person relationship as the bond with the mother grows and becomes mutually supportive. It goes on then to become a three-person relationship with the introduction of a second adult, usually the father, but not always, and that is then a family relationship. The child goes on from there to form relationships with the wider group of people, probably including nursery and eventually school, and that is them functioning in the outside world. Winnicott describes this process in significant detail, and includes thoughts and ideas of what happens if things go wrong. In his book, *Home is where we start from* (Winnicott and Winnicott, 1990) he gives lots of examples of the impact of different home environments and experiences. In his book *Deprivation and Delinquency* (Winnicott, 1985), he charts the processes that a child will go through in situations of emotional deprivation (and physical deprivation) that becomes the forerunners to delinquent behaviour. This we now see as trauma-related behaviour that challenges in people with additional intellectual disabilities. It is very clear from Winnicott's work that we can see how particular early experiences have a traumatic impact on the development of the personality, and how these impact on who the adult becomes.

John Bowlby was the first person who made a foray into the world of attachment. His book is now called *the secure base* and was originally *the making and breaking of affectional bonds* (Bowlby, 1988). Bowlby describes the process of the development of attachment between child and adult. He does not put as much emphasis as Winnicott on the need for this to be the mother. He makes clear that children will make attachments to the person who is close, proximal, and meets the needs in a reliable and affectionate way. He also brought to the attention of the general public the effect of separation from the attachment figure. This was demonstrated very much in his observation of children who were hospitalised. Prior to his intervention, it had been believed, that children who became distressed when hospitalised were better if they didn't see their parents and would settle down to the ward routine more quickly. What Bowlby pointed out was that in fact the children initially made a protest when left, and that when they became quiet, they were in fact traumatised and shut down, and some of them would struggle to recover from this. So, it was Bowlby who first introduced open visiting for children in hospital. It is difficult to think about this now as something that was policy, when we clearly have the ability of parents to stay in hospital with their children. That was how it was and at the time people believed they were doing the right thing. Bowlby coined the term 'pathological mourning' for the condition of some children who gave up hope that their attachment figure was coming back for them and we can see this as the forerunner of endogenous depression.

Melanie Klein is considered quite difficult to read and I would agree with that. There is also some criticism that her research was based on her own children (Grosskurth, 1986). However, she gives us some useful insights into early emotional development. The first is that she emphasises the fact that the relationship with the child begins in the womb, not at the time of delivery. She puts a great deal of emphasis on the need for that relationship to be warm and supportive throughout the developmental period. She talks particularly about something she calls the 'depressive position' (Klein, 1980), which is that point in development where the child comes to accept that the parent can be both good and bad, can provide and meet needs, can also take away. People who do not reach the depressive position, that point of acceptance of the positive and negative in their attachment figures, are the ones who do not reach the psychological birth referred to by Mahler. The advantage of the Mahler work is that the observable behaviours can be measured. Klein's work is not so easy to transfer into a tool that is useful across a wide range of people.

These three key psychoanalysts, Winnicott, Bowlby and Klein, gave us a real insight into early development. None of them were working with children with intellectual disabilities. Mahler was not particularly working with children with intellectual disabilities, although some of her cohort probably did have some limitations. So, my work has taken from all four of them, with some additional factors from Freud, to arrive at a way of understanding, observing and measuring the emotional development, so that we can see when things have gone wrong. We can recognise that what has gone wrong has been traumatic, and, by measuring the stage of development, we can work out what type of trauma and when it is likely to have occurred. This gives us the possibility of therapeutic intervention. People who do not have ID but have gone through the traumatic experiences of early childhood that have affected their attachment and emotional security, will almost certainly have recognisable mental health issues. At its most extreme, with trauma before the age of one, there will be serious personality disorders and psychotic illnesses. With people who have experienced trauma between one and three, there may be varying levels of depression, anxiety, dissociation, and erratic behaviour linked with their insecure sense of self.

Babies and children with intellectual disabilities have a range of experiences to contend with over and above what they would have had if they did not have an ID. They may have started life in intensive care, they may be a twin, they may have suffered birth injuries, and there may be a range of reasons why they have an ID. Some of those reasons will have led to traumatic events that are designed to help them, and do help them physically, sometimes to keep them alive. But, by their very nature, they are likely to have interfered with their emotional development. If we take, for example, the need for close attachment in very early childhood, then we can see the need for intensive care will interfere with the process. If they must have surgery and be separated from their primary carer that will also be traumatic. As they move into the toddler stage, if they have limited mobility, they may be left alone in one part of the house while mum gets on with work in another part of the house, because she knows the child will not get up to mischief. But if the child cannot keep in mind that mum will come back then it will become distressed and, after a time, may shut down in the way that Bowlby spoke about. One of the big issues that comes up is the one of secondary carers. Because of the need to stimulate cognitive development as soon as possible in children with intellectual disabilities, there is a tendency for them to go to nursery and playgroup early. If they are not emotionally ready for that separation this again can cause distress. If it is recognised that they are not able to maintain a sense of self at the age of three or four when most children will achieve this, it is possible to put in place an attachment programme whereby when the child is transferred from mum to carer it is done formally with no gaps. So, the child who travels to nursery on the bus is transferred from mum to the escort, then from the escort to the school staff in a very formal way so that the child is never left feeling who is there for them. Putting this in place has quite miraculous results in many cases. The child is then able to engage in the stimulating activity that is provided, secure in the knowledge that they are safe, and anxiety becomes manageable.

I have tried in this chapter to summarise the work of many years. As a clinical psychologist, trained scientifically to use data and research findings, it is sometimes difficult to accept the writings of psychoanalysts, whose work is not measured and usually cannot be easily replicated. Having always had an interest in psychodynamic psychotherapy, and what the analysts say, I sought at an early stage of my career to find a path that incorporated both science and subjective experience. Finding Mahler's work gave me that way in, where the observable behaviour that represented stages of emotional development could be measured. What I have also found (Frankish, 2016) is that most psychotherapy with people with disabilities is based on trauma that occurred in early life, before the formation of a sense of self. Most psychotherapy with people without disabilities, but not all, is based on events that have been intellectually processed, and therefore happened after the development and establishment of a sense of self. It does mean that therapy with this client group must be provided from a position of being able to tolerate the pain of the immature, emotional self. This requires long-term psychotherapy and is not usually readily available, especially not on the National Health Service. Having a model of understanding the behavioural consequences of early trauma allows us to provide training for support staff to provide an emotionally nurturing environment. This provides a developmental opportunity for children and adults with intellectual disabilities. And that developmental opportunity allows them to grow emotionally and gradually to facilitate the emotional development to be in tune with their cognitive development. In my clinical work I have seen this work dramatically and it is reassuring, both that the theory is correct, and that lives can be significantly improved. The book *'Disability Psychotherapy – An Innovative Approach to Trauma Informed Care'*, gives a more detailed explanation of the theory and examples of the application (Frankish, 2016).

References

Balint M (1979) *The Basic Fault: Therapeutic aspects of regression*. London: Taylor Francis.

Bowlby J (1988) *The Secure Base*. London: Routledge.

Frankish P (1989) Meeting the emotional needs of handicapped people: a psychodynamic approach. *Journal of Mental Deficiency Research* **33** 407–414.

Frankish P (2003) *The influence of developmental trauma on behaviour in adults with a learning disability*. Doctoral thesis. University of Hull

Frankish P (2016) *Disability Psychotherapy: An innovative approach to trauma-informed care*. London: Karnac

Freud S (1895) *Studies in Hysteria*. Standard Edition, 2. London: Hogarth.

Grosskurth P (1986) *Melanie Klein: Her world and her work* London: Jason Aronson Inc.

Klein M (1980) Envy and Gratitude: and other works (1946-1963). London: Virago Press.

Mahler M, Pine F, & Bergman A., (1975 reprinted 2000) *The Psychological Birth of The Human Infant*. New York: Basic Books.

Winnicott DW (1964) *The Child, the Family and the Outside World*. Harmondsworth: Penguin.

Winnicott DW (1985) *Deprivation and Delinquency*. London: Routledge.

Winnicott DW & Winnicott C (1990) *Home is where we start from*. Harmondsworth: Penguin.

Chapter 6:
Finding out about trauma in the lives of people with intellectual disabilities; and what to do about it

Allan Skelly

'There is no greater agony than bearing an untold story inside you.'
– Maya Angelou

This chapter explores:

- psychological trauma (and how new traumas are worsened by earlier or chronic trauma)
- how trauma affects people with IDs
- what may indicate the presence of trauma
- how psychological assessment can be helpful
- the nature of attachment behavioural strategies and what happens when these no longer work
- how attachment interventions both by specialists, and carers in general, can help.

A self-report rating scale is presented, which may be helpful for clients, carers and professionals working in partnership to address trauma and attachment issues.

What is trauma and how does trauma affect people?

For the purposes of this chapter, trauma refers to the experience of a shocking or distressing event(s) that overwhelms the person's ability to cope. The additional meaning of physical injury as used in medicine, is not used here.

Discrete trauma when a person was loved, supported and comforted as a child, will nonetheless overcome coping mechanisms when it is extreme, such as with combat veterans, or survivors of road-traffic collisions. Typically, the person tries to forget the experience, only to be visited by distressing memories, which occur involuntarily. They avoid anything that reminds them of the trauma (triggers), but this can cause practical problems or unreasonable fears. This is sometimes referred to as a post-traumatic syndrome or stress disorder (PTS or PTSD). While PTS based on a single experience can need psychological treatment, it is possible to reduce its effects in relatively straightforward ways such as graded exposure to triggers (gradually learning not to avoid feared situations), or Eye Movement Desensitisation and Reprocessing (EMDR) , which stops the person trying to push down memories, leading them to eventually lose their power. However, people with moderate to profound ID may not be able to engage in such sessions because language skills are required. Yet, some evidence for these approaches shows promise in people with mild to moderate ID (Mivessen *et al.*, 2016), with several positive case reports. A psychologist working in community services for people who have intellectual disabilities should be able to provide this treatment or refer to a colleague who can.

Sadly, many referrals for psychological help are for individuals who have experienced repeated, multiple and significant traumas. A commonly used measure of these is the adverse childhood experiences (ACEs) checklist. The effect of ACEs on health are well demonstrated in general populations that present to their family practitioner (Felitti *et al.*, 1998). These include: a higher risk of alcohol or drug problems; low mood; high rates of heart and lung disease; aggressive histories; vulnerability to violence; and higher likelihood of imprisonment. ACEs include: emotional, physical or sexual abuse; neglect; growing up where adults have alcohol, drug or mental health problems; where there is domestic violence; an incarcerated adult; or where parents have split up. ACEs do not include poverty, bullying at school, or bereavements, though these are also known to be important traumas that affect later psychological health as well.

We do know that children with intellectual disabilities are at much greater risk of such experiences than other children. For example, a large population-based study in Sussex found that children with moderate to severe ID were more likely to be registered for child protection; 2.9 times more likely to be registered for emotional abuse; 3.4 times more for physical abuse, 5.3 times more for neglect; and 6.4 times more for sexual abuse (Spencer *et al.*, 2005). Similar 'multiplied' levels of maltreatment have been found in the USA (Sullivan and Knutson, 2000; McDonnell *et al.*, 2019), Canada (Dion *et al.*, 2018) and in Australia (Mclean *et al.*, 2017). We also know that women with ID are at higher risk of unwanted sexual activity and/or assault from partners (Martin at al, 2006), and that a high number of care staff will anonymously admit to assaulting people with ID in their care (Strand *et al.*, 2004).

Latrogenic trauma occurs when professionals or services unconsciously or unavoidably undertake actions that introduce trauma or worsen the effects of previous trauma. Since the impact of caring for a child with an intellectual disability (ID) can be stressful, some of the raised risk of the above maltreatment occurs because families are under pressure. The Joseph Rountree Foundation (2001) found that the financial cost alone of caring for a child with a disability was on average double that of caring for a non-disabled child. But services can seem detached and this can hurt family carers.

'I don't want any other mother to have to go through what I did. To sit in office after office and listen to doctors, social workers, all of them, talk about me and my child as if we weren't real. We have feelings.'
– Mother of young child with ID

The same report found evidence that professionals can ask personal questions insensitively, that there are repeated assessments but much less support and intervention, and that building up a long-term relationship with a particular professional was unlikely. Some professionals would refer to them as a '[Disability x] family'. At other times they felt completely ignored (readers may find this ironic, given what we know about attachment theory – see below). Despite the heightened risks, many if not most families adjust to the needs of their child where they can remain within family care.

Some people will require periods of specialised care that cannot be provided at home. Perhaps the most traumatic experience for people with ID is admission to hospital after a physical, behavioural or mental health crisis. People with ID tend to have poorer experience of hospital and worse outcomes (Iacono *et al.*, 2014), and families can be distressed by separation and loss of influence over the decisions made for the person. In the UK, there is also a higher risk of being maltreated within assessment and treatment (A&T) units, as revealed by repeated scandals (BBC News, 25th May 2019). Institutions then, perhaps by their very nature, promote maltreatment that introduces, or worsens, psychological trauma, at a time when the person is especially vulnerable, and their family have broken or non-existent access to them. Therefore, the UK government is committed to end the use of hospital care for people with ID who have behavioural or mental health difficulties, though progress is slow and there are complex challenges in the system (Voluntary Organisations Disability Group, 2018).

Noticing the signs of trauma where the person cannot directly express it

Those who can express the trauma and who have someone who will truly listen; share their experiences by describing it in a 'narrative'. Merely starting to share negative experiences – relatively easy for most – involves complex psychological skills. One must find a safe person and safe place to tell them, to be able to name the emotion, and describe it to the other person in a way they can understand. Add to that the serious and difficult task of overcoming trauma, which involves remembering it clearly and in sequence, tolerating frightening feelings, rediscovering the successful survival, and restoring faith in one's everyday safety. Many people with severe and profound ID will not be able to transform their experience into words and may require the kind of tentative and uncertain understanding of their state of mind that new parents have to guess.

Those with experience of caring for or working with people with ID will be aware that their life history is often chequered. Signs of a trauma reaction can be recognised, and include:

- frequent memories and talk of adverse experiences (trauma events)
- bad dreams and disturbed sleep
- physical or emotional symptoms when reminded of the experiences
- extreme reactions to low-threat situations
- loss of reasoning
- irritability
- panic
- desperately attempting to escape a situation even when safe
- hyperventilation (over-breathing)
- aggression
- difficulty concentrating
- clinging to a significant other

- watchfulness
- lack of trust in others
- avoidance of services
- disengaging from support/approach-avoid
- using alcohol or drugs to block out memories.

Of course, some of these signs do not necessarily imply trauma, and so corroborating facts will be needed during any investigation. The list is certainly not exhaustive. Carers will also be aware that when these signs are present – they will feel the need to address the problem by understanding why it has occurred. They may, therefore, move towards the person in order to help, when it is by no means clear if this will reassure the person or exacerbate their distress.

Therefore, it is a distinct possibility that people with ID presenting to services for help with behavioural or emotional difficulties may have experienced a recent trauma that re-triggers their earlier trauma responses. This can seem like aggression, which obtains attention or escape. Self-injury may be a self-distraction technique that also communicates the need for help; compulsive behaviour may be an attempt to manage extreme anxiety or loneliness; neglecting one's personal care may reflect low self-esteem due to past emotional abuse; and so on.

While behavioural difficulties will usually be assessed by way of a behavioural functional analysis, carers and families should feel able to voice concerns about past trauma, and its potential effects on behaviours. It is written into policy in the UK that trauma and maltreatment should be included in these assessments (NICE, 2015a).

Since it is hard to tell – how might trauma be more formally assessed in people with ID?

In the UK, carers and families are welcome to make a referral for more specialist help through their family doctor. There should be a psychological service available either through a specialist mental health team making adjustments for the person's disability, or by the local specialist team for people who have ID, who will have a psychologist among their team.

As one might expect, there is a problem of using self-report scales designed for people without ID, such as the Impact of Events Scale, which is often used in services designed to help with PTSD.

A psychological assessment may therefore involve observations, interviews with carers, meeting the person, and taking a clear history. There are two scales designed specifically for people with ID; the Impact of Events Scale-Intellectual Disabilities (IES-ID; Hall *et al.,* 2014) and the Lancaster and Northgate Trauma Scale (LANTS; Wigham *et al.,* 2011). They involve a series of questions in interview style, making them suitable for people with mild to moderate IDs, who can understand the questions. The scales are scientifically reliable and appear to measure trauma (and some other aspects of distress), although they need to be researched further. The LANTS also includes an informant-based scale for people who cannot self-report, which tends to correlate with disturbances of behaviours that carers can code on a scale (for example, the Behaviour Problems Inventory, Rojahn, *et al.* 2012a; 2012b).

Such assessments can lead to a psychological formulation, which explains how the signs of can be an unsatisfactory way for the person to express that they are still distressed. For people whose trauma is longstanding and reflects serious maltreatment as a child, it is necessary to consider how they interact with those closest to them emotionally, as this will be crucial in deciding how to move forward.

Attachment theory – and how it can help

One important aspect of human interaction is how emotional communication in relationships can help us heal deep distress, such as that which flows from the experience of ACEs and other significant traumas.

'I once said: "there is no such thing as an infant", meaning of course, that whenever one finds an infant one finds [parental] care, and without [parental] care there would be no infant.'

– Donald Winnicott

Winnicott's ideas gained support when attachment theory was developed by John Bowlby, who had discovered deep psychological problems in poorly cared-for orphans who had been caught stealing (Bowlby, 1946). Attachment theory suggests that high-quality early care based in a reliable and close emotional bond is essential for healthy psychological development. The theory has now been extensively researched and supported, but people with ID are usually excluded from both research and policy. This might seem strange, given that children with ID who are subject to child protection may be three times more likely to have marked difficulties in attachment than children without disabilities who require protection (Dion *et al.,* 2018). Several publications provide more detailed information on how this can be addressed (British Psychological Society, 2017; Fletcher *et al.,* 2016).

Most people achieve autonomy through consistent childhood experiences of safety, encouragement to play and explore, their parents' delight in their creative play, and comforting at times of stress or hurt. The parent should respond to the child's distress by welcoming, reassuring, and by giving words, and therefore meaning, to painful emotions. As the caregiver behavioural system becomes attuned to the attachment behavioural system of the child, the child learns how to label pain and upsetting feelings, which also provides a reassuring limit to it, as the parent can 'make it better'. Through difficulties that are due to communication issues, or maltreatment, a person with ID may struggle to gain the resulting feeling that parents (and authority in general) can be trusted to support their learning and be around to help if things become difficult. We do know that it is relatively difficult for parents of children with Down's Syndrome to understand the intonation of their cries (Cicchetti and Serafica, 1981). Some children with complex physical difficulties or chronic illnesses, especially when painful, may have limited experiences of satisfying relaxation.

However, ACEs by their nature involve problems in the care provided to the child and people with ID are therefore at increased risk of attachment difficulties. It is known that where autonomy is not achieved, the children with ID are more likely to show attachment that is more typical of severely maltreated children (British Psychological Society, 2017).

Mary Ainsworth and colleagues (Ainsworth *et al.*, 1978) famously determined how attachment insecurity develops in very young children, using the strange situation (SS). The SS involves the parent leaving the room while the child is playing; an adult stranger enters the room; then the parent returns. How the child and parent interact will determine whether the child is secure (happy to see parent; re-engaging in play; joyfully), avoidant (e.g. turning away from the parent; as though comforting is not needed; parent rebuffing approach from the child), or resistant (very upset on separation; difficulty in settling; parent is intermittently engaged or 'unavailable'). This simple technique determines behavioural patterns that correspond to the person's later internal state of mind with a surprising amount of stability across the lifetime, although security can be developed at any stage in most people who start off with avoidant or resistant patterns.

Later, Mary Main (Main and Solomon, 1990) noted that children with more severe experiences of trauma, or whose parents were deeply grieving, showed signs of a breakdown of attachment strategies, a terrified state of mind, or 'fright without solution'. This often implies maltreatment (though not necessarily) and may therefore be of interest to child protection services, as the child is watchful and may 'freeze' in response to the return of the parent in the SS.

In adults, the corresponding states of mind to each category of child behaviour are often referred to with the terms in Table 1. These were carefully identified by the scientific work of Carol George and her colleagues, using a method called the adult attachment interview (AAI; George *et al.*, 1985). Unfortunately, the method requires rigorous training and expert techniques, and one feature of responses, 'incoherence', can be confused with the cognitive limitations of ID itself. Therefore, the AAI is not used by clinicians to assess attachment in adults with ID, even though they are likely to demonstrate the same categories of attachment behaviours.

Table 1: Categories of Attachment

Child category	Adult state of mind
Insecure-avoidant	Dismissing
Secure	Autonomous
Insecure-ambivalent	Preoccupied
Disorganised	Unresolved

Signs of disturbances in attachment will depend on the person's attachment behavioural system. If the person expects their care to be supportive, available, and empathic, they will be more likely to overcome even serious early trauma, because they will be more able to re-establish trust in the world and other people.

However, if they expect those who care for them to be irritable, hostile, and to minimise their distress, they may develop a dismissing attachment behavioural system, where they avoid others at times of stress or express their distress indirectly, or through behaviours. For example, a young man living in a shared home felt angry about the care and attention given to other clients, while coming to terms with the death of a family member. He began to leave urine in cups around the home. When questioned about this, he became extremely angry and threatening, and ran out of the room.

Conversely, if a person expects those who care for them to be warm and helpful some of the time, but at other times to be withdrawn, inexpressive or demanding, then they may develop a preoccupied attachment behavioural system. For example, a young woman subjected to repeated instances of physical abuse from a former boyfriend became highly concerned about her care team's rota, and was considered very 'clingy' and focused on preferred staff to work with her. When the team were rotated to limit contact of preferred staff with her, her mental health deteriorated and she was assessed for detention under mental health legislation, after becoming confused and terrified, and convinced that her ex-partner had arranged for the change in staff approach.

Note that in this last example, the person whose attachment needs were not addressed began to show signs of 'fright without solution' (the disorganisation of attachment). This unresolved relating is noted when one of the other categories is present for some of the time and, unlike the other classification categories, is not considered mutually exclusive.

How can a person's attachment be assessed more formally?

It is possible for professionals to assess attachment more formally in people with ID, but it is important for carers and families to consult with professionals who have formal training in attachment theory. The very accessibility of attachment-based ideas has made it both a useful way of considering the care of children who may be at risk, and of promoting the physical and emotional security of children in interventions. Attachment-based interventions are known to be highly effective in children within the care system (NICE, 2015b).

However, a little knowledge can be dangerous. There are several concepts utilising Bowlby's original idea, and they are not entirely the same thing.

- Attachment behaviours: the seeking and maintaining of proximity to achieve protection and support e.g. proximity seeking, contact maintaining, avoiding, resisting, disorganisation of these. As observed in the SS.

- Attachment relationship: description of the dyadic history of attachment behaviour and response.

- Attachment bond: affective concern with a relationship perceived as stable, including desire for contact, dislike of separation and the need for comfort during separation.

- Attachment representation: unconscious internal rules relating to attachment e.g. coded as avoidant / dismissing, autonomous / secure, anxious / preoccupied, disorganised / unresolved. As seen in the AAI.

- Attachment style: the internal judgement that one feels comfortable getting close to others, and depending on them, or not: comfortable with intimacy and autonomy (secure), preoccupied with relationships, dismissing of intimacy and fiercely independent, or fearful of intimacy and actively avoidant. As seen in questionnaires about romantic relationships in adults.

■ Attachment disorder: specific patterns of atypical behaviours in the context of pathogenic care: inhibited, withdrawn, or indiscriminately social. As used by psychiatric professionals seeking a formal diagnosis of mental conditions.

In fact, it is rare for rigorous coding of behaviour to be used in ID services by way of the SS, or the rigorous observational method of the adult attachment projective (AAP), even though they have been used in research (Bhakar *et al.*, 2018). Professionals will often choose self-report or informant-based scales, which are much more brief and non-intrusive, and are therefore easily integrated into assessment sessions. Examples of this include the secure base safe haven observation checklist (SBSHO), a scale containing 20 quick item ratings on seven-point scales. This scale can help predict certain forms of behaviours that challenge, identifying children who may need help (de Schipper and Schuengel, 2010).

The Manchester Attachment Scale – Third-party measure (MAS-T) has only 16 judgements on four-point scales and is designed to be filled in by an informant, such as a carer who knows the person well. Designed to screen people with all levels of ID for non-secure attachment, this scale also shows some prediction of behaviours that challenge (Penketh *et al.*, 2013).

A third example of such a scale is the quality of early relatedness rating scale (QuERRS), an 18-item scale containing judgements on five-point scales. The QuERRS was originally designed to help psychotherapists to understand their clients' internal representations of their attachments in childhood. The scale can predict the need for more sessions of therapy in people with mild to moderate ID, and features of the case indicating high or low levels of severity (Skelly and Harvey, 2017). The scale has now been subject to analysis of more than 100 cases, which has allowed it to be tested for how it matches up to the predictions of attachment theory. Interestingly, hostile incoherence and security appear to be opposite poles, suggesting that low hostility or dismissing attachment goes with having a clear story about one's past. Interpersonal pain scores reflect disorganisation of attachment, and fearful preoccupation relates to preoccupied attachments in the person's mind (Skelly *et al.*, 2019).

A self-report version of the QuERRS (sQuERRS) is shown at the end of the chapter for illustrative purposes. It could be administered by a carer who would support or scaffold the client to give one of the five responses to each statement (not true at all, only a little, half-true or sometimes, mostly true, or completely true). There is also a guide to the meaning of the three scores produced. It is recommended that a psychologist or psychotherapist with formal training in attachment theory is consulted when interpreting the results for more than just personal interest. Carers should also remember that such procedures can only be done with informed consent and confidentiality, and results should not be shared with third parties unless the person gives permission.

Other procedures have been developed for use with people with intellectual disabilities, including the clinical observation of attachment (COA), which has been used with children who have ID (Boris *et al.*, 2007), and a modified choice description method for assessment of romantic attachment style (Larson *et al.*, 2011).

A word on interventions; should we be optimistic about how attachment can help overcome trauma in people with ID?

There is reason to be optimistic about attachment-based interventions. There are specialist interventions with more than one study demonstrating success:

- Psychological therapy with a focus on attachments and trauma recovery, such as disability psychotherapy (Frankish, 1989), psychodynamic therapy (Skelly *et al.*, 2018); or cognitive analytic therapy (CAT; Beard *et al.*, 2016)

- Video interaction guidance and feedback: a method of carer feedback using short, repeated video feedback sessions, which aim to improve attunement in the caregiver behavioural system. This has been demonstrated with people with ID in the Netherlands (Damen *et al.*, 2011)

- For children with multiple disabilities including visual impairment and intellectual disabilities, integrative therapy for attachment and behaviour has been shown to have the potential for better results than behavioural interventions alone (Schuengel *et al.*, 2009).

These interventions are provided by specialists on referral to highly skilled teams and are not yet widely accessible to those providing everyday care. Video interaction guidance is widely used in children's services, such as looked after children's (LAC) services, and it is to be hoped that it will become more widely available in services for people who have intellectual disabilities and care teams.

However, attachment-based interventions can be seen as a set of principles to incorporate into all forms of caring. For example, the SECURED intervention (Skelly, 2018) is a relatively simple model for parents and carers, which is based on the same essential principles as the SBSHO method. Carers are encouraged to provide Safety, Empathy, Consistency of presence (as opposed to multiple carers), Unconditional regard, Realism about the person's emotional and cognitive development, supporting Exploration of new learning and experiences, and Delighting in the person. It is also expected that the person can seek support from the carer when in distressed and be helped to understand it.

Models like the SECURED approach can be seen as a set of principles and a user-friendly understanding of attachment theory where practices that are contrary to emotional well-being can be challenged within caring organisations and families themselves. For example, sudden changes in placements can be discouraged; sudden changes in personnel can be minimised; losses of trusted carers acknowledged as a potential cause of trauma; placement permanence and deep, enduring relationships can be valued as goals in themselves. In doing so, we might be able to hope that the outcomes sought for people with ID include intimacy, friendship, shared enjoyable experiences, and love, as well as the current focus on the reduction of behavioural or mental health symptoms.

The usual rites of passage are also sometimes denied to people with ID. We know that they are often excluded from family funerals, celebrations or other events on grounds of behaviour, or a misguided idea that they might be confused or upset. Again, a trauma- and attachment-aware care system would not allow for such exclusions, because trauma needs to be acknowledged, shared and processed, in the context of a safe and trusting relationship.

Conclusions

'The big issue for traumatised people is that they don't own themselves ... And so what we have learned is what makes you resilient to trauma is to own yourself fully.'
– Bessel van der Kolk, The Body Keeps the Score

There is clearly a huge health inequality whereby children with intellectual disabilities are known to be at risk but do not receive services that would help them (Wigham and Emerson, 2015). It is surely unacceptable that the most deserving should be the least served; that those asked to struggle uphill in life should also be subject to unnecessary slings and arrows. Let there be testament to their agonies; facts revealed, their thoughts and feelings heard, understood and shared.

Recognising trauma and getting it formally assessed helps us consider together how to put words to such things, at all levels of society and in all our working and personal relationships. In doing so, we allow a person to take back some control of their own mind and body. In one's attachments, we seek to achieve a sense that there is freedom to safely enjoy life's rich experiences with others – and to know that comfort and support is available, when a shoulder to cry on, or something more, is needed.

Resource note

Kind permission for appropriately trained personnel to obtain the LANTS via email contact has been provided by Professor John Taylor (john.taylor@cntw.nhs.uk) and Dr Sarah Wigham (Sarah.Wigham@newcastle.ac.uk).

The QuERRS-2 for practitioners such as psychologists or psychotherapists is available by corresponding with the author at allan.skelly@cntw.nhs.uk

©The sQuERRS is the intellectual property of Cumbria, Northumberland, Tyne & Wear NHS Foundation Trust. Suitably qualified persons may make copies of the scales for clinical use. The sQuERRS is printed for demonstrative purposes. If carers support a person with ID to complete a sQuERRS on the advice of a professional such as a psychologist, it is strongly advised that the results are interpreted by a similarly qualified clinician with psychometric competency. For further advice, or to register for research use, please contact allan.skelly@cntw.nhs.uk.

References

Ainsworth MD, Blehar M, Waters, E & Wall S (1978) *Patterns of Attachment: A psychological study of the strange situation* Hillsdale, New Jersey: Lawrence Erlbaum.

BBC News (22 May 2019) *Whorlton Hall: Hospital 'Abused' Vulnerable Adults* [online]. Available at: bbc. co.uk

Beard K, Greenhill B & Lloyd J (2016) Cognitive analytic therapy. In: N Beail (Ed) *Psychological Therapies and People with Intellectual Disabilities*. Leicester: UK; British Psychological Society.

Bhaker R, Clegg JA, Bell B & Schuengel C (2013) *A reliability study of the Reunion Coding Scheme for the Strange Situation for adults with severe intellectual disabilities*. New Horizons for Mental Health in Intellectual & Developmental Disabilities: 9th congress of the European Congress of Mental Health in Intellectual Disabilities. Lisbon, Portugal.

Boris NW, Fueyo M & Zeanah CH (2007) The clinical assessment of attachment in children under five. *Journal of the American Academy of Child and Adolescent Psychiatry* **36** (2) 291–293.

Bowlby J (1946) *Forty-four Juvenile Thieves: Their character and home-life*. Baillere: Tindall & Cox.

British Psychological Society (2017) *Incorporating Attachment Theory into Practice: Clinical practice guideline for clinical psychologists working with people with intellectual disabilities*. Leicester, UK: BPS publications.

Cicchetti D & Serafica FC (1981) Interplay among behavioural systems: illustrations from the study of attachment, affiliation, and wariness in young-children with Downs syndrome. *Developmental Psychology* **17** 36–49.

Damen S, Kef S, Worm M, Janssen MJ & Schuengel C (2011) Effects of video-feedback interaction training for professional caregivers of children and adults with visual and intellectual disabilities. *Journal of Intellectual Disability Research* **55** 581–595.

de Schipper JC & Schuengel C (2010) Attachment behaviour towards support staff in young people with intellectual disabilities: associations with challenging behaviour. *Journal of Intellectual Disability Research* **54** (7) 584–596.

Dion J, Paquette G, Tremblay K-N, Collin-Vezina D, Chabot M (2018) Child maltreatment among children with intellectual disability in the Canadian Incidence Study. *American Journal on Intellectual and Developmental Disabilities* **123** (2) 176–188.

Felitti VJ, Anda RF, Nordenberg D, Williamson DF, Spitz AM, Edwards V & Marks JS (1998) Relationship of childhood abuse and household dysfunction to many of the leading causes of death in adults: The Adverse Childhood Experiences (ACE) Study. *American Journal of Preventative Medicine* **14** 245–258.

Fletcher H, Flood A & Hare D (2016) *Attachment in Intellectual and Developmental Disability: A clinician's guide to practice and research*. New York: Wiley.

Frankish P (1989) Meeting the emotional needs of handicapped people: A psycho-dynamic approach. *Journal of Mental Deficiency Research* **33** 407–414.

George C, Kaplan N, & Main M (1985) *Adult Attachment Interview Protocol* (3rd edition). Berkeley, USA: University of California.

Hall JC, Jobson L & Langdon PE (2014) Measuring symptoms of post-traumatic stress disorder in people with intellectual disabilities: The development and psychometric properties of the Impact of Event Scale-Intellectual Disabilities (IES-ID). *British Journal of Clinical Psychology* **53** (3) 315–332.

Iocono T, Bigby C, Unsworth C, Douglas J & Fitzpatrick P (2014) A systematic review of hospital experiences of people with intellectual disability. *BMC Health Services Research* **14** 505.

Joseph Rountree Foundation (2001) *The Impact of Childhood Disability on Family Life*. York, UK: York Publishing Services ltd.

Larson F, Alim N & Tsakanikos E (2011) Attachment style and mental health in adults with intellectual disability: self-reports and reports by carers. *Advances in Mental Health and Intellectual Disabilities* **5** 15–23.

Main M & Solomon J (1990) Procedures for identifying infants as disorganised/disoriented during the Ainsworth Strange Situation. In: Greenberg MT, Cicchetti D, Cummings, EM (Eds), *Attachment in the Preschool Years*. University of Chicago Press, Chicago, IL, USA, pp. 121–160.

Martin SL, Ray N, Sotres-Alvarez D, Kupper LL, Moracco KE, Dickens PA, Scandlin D & Gizlice Z (2006) Physical and sexual assault of women with disabilities. *Violence Against Women* **12** (9) 823–37.

McDonnell CG, Boan, AD, Bradley, CC, Seay KD, Charles, JM & Carpenter, LA (2019) Child maltreatment in autism spectrum disorder and intellectual disability: results from a population-based study. *Journal of Child Psychology and Psychiatry* **60** (5) 576–584.

Mclean MJ, Sims S, Bower C, Leonard H, Stanley FJ & O'Donnell M (2017) Maltreatment risk among children with disabilities. *Pediatrics* **130** (4) e20161817.

Mivessen L, Didden R & de Jongh A (2016) *Assessment and Treatment of PTSD in People with Intellectual Disabilities: Comprehensive guide to post-traumatic stress disorder*. Switzerland: Springer.

National Institute for Health and Care Excellence (NICE; 2015a) *Challenging Behaviour and Learning Disabilities: Prevention and interventions for people with learning disabilities whose behaviour challenges* [online]. Available at: nice.org.uk.

National Institute for Health and Clinical Excellence (NICE; 2015b) *Children's Attachment: Attachment in children and young people who are adopted from care, in care or at high risk of going into care* [online]. Available at nice.org.uk.

Penketh V, Walker S, Flood A, Hendy S & Hare DJ (2013) Attachment in adults with intellectual disabilities: The examination of the psychometric properties of the Manchester Attachment Scale- Third Party Observational Measure (MAST). *Journal of Applied Research in Intellectual Disabilities*, **27** (5) 458-470.

Rojahn J, Rowe EW, Sharber AC, Hastings RP, Matson JL, Didden R, Kroes DBH & Dumont ELM (2012a) The Behavior Problems Inventory-Short Form (BPI-S) for individuals with intellectual disabilities I: Development and provisional clinical reference data. *Journal of Intellectual Disability Research* **56**, 527–545.

Rojahn J, Rowe EW, Sharber AC, Hastings RP, Matson JL, Didden R, Kroes DBH & Dumont ELM (2012b) The Behavior Problems Inventory-Short Form (BPI-S) for individuals with intellectual disabilities II: Reliability and Validity. *Journal of Intellectual Disability Research* **56**, 546–565.

Schuengel C, Sterkenburg PS, Jeczynski P, Janssen CGC & Jongbloed G (2009) Supporting affect regulation in children with multiple disabilities during psychotherapy: A multiple case design study of therapeutic attachment. *Journal of Consulting and Clinical Psychology* **77** 291–301.

Skelly A (2018) Trauma-informed practice in intellectual disability services: Recommendations for mental health professionals in the UK. *Bulletin of the Faculty for People with Intellectual Disabilities of the British Psychological Society* **16** (1) 13-17.

Skelly A & Harvey H (2017) Attachment representations in psychological therapy of people with intellectual disabilities; a preliminary factor analytic study of the Quality of Early Relationships Rating Scale (QuERRS). *Bulletin of the Faculty for People with Intellectual Disabilities of the British Psychological Society* **15** (1) 32–37.

Skelly A, McGeehan C & Usher R (2018) An open trial of psychodynamic psychotherapy for people with mild-moderate intellectual disabilities with waiting list and follow up control. *Advances in Mental Health and Intellectual Disabilities* **12** (5/6) 153–162.

Skelly A, Windebank P & Usher R (2019) *Therapist rating scale of attachment representations in psychological therapy of people with intellectual disabilities: factor analysis of the QuERRS-2.* Proceedings of the Annual Conference of the Faculty for People with Intellectual Disabilities of the British Psychological Society. London, 2-3 April 2019.

Spencer N, Devereux E, Wallace A, Sundrum R, Shenoy M, Bacchus C & Logan S (2005) Disabling conditions and registration for child abuse and neglect: A population-based study. *Paediatrics* **116** (3) 609–14.

Strand M, Benzein E & Saveman BI (2004) Violence in the care of adult persons with intellectual disabilities. *Journal of Clinical Nursing* **13** (4) 506–14.

Wigham S & Emerson E (2015) Trauma and life events in adults with intellectual disability. *Current Developmental Disorders Report* **2** (2) 93–99.

Wigham S, Hatton C & Taylor JL (2011) The Lancaster and Northgate Trauma Scales (LANTS): The development and psychometric properties of a measure of trauma for people with mild to moderate intellectual disabilities. *Research in Developmental Disabilities* **32** 2651–2659.

Voluntary Organisations Disability Group (2018) *Transforming Care: The challenges and solutions* London, UK: VODG publications.

Appendix 1: self-rated Quality of Interpersonal Relatedness Rating Scale (sQuERRS)

Self-rated Quality of Early Relatedness Rating Scale (sQuERRS)

Person's ID: / Date:	Instructions for administration: Please read or listen to the item, then rate how 'true for me' the statement is.	Not true at all	Only a little true	Half true, or sometimes	Mostly true	Very true	HI	IP	FP
		PLEASE circle the correct rating. One score only for each statement. Untrue ←---→ Very true					OFFICE USE ONLY		
1	I don't remember much about my childhood. It didn't affect me.	0	1	2	3	4			
2	I'm realistic about my childhood and its effect on me.	4	3	2	1	0			
3	I had to look after one or both parents when they weren't well – emotionally, physically or both.	0	1	2	3	4			
4	I was hurt a lot as a child. This is still affecting my feelings.	0	1	2	3	4			
5 optional	I might be safe now, but I don't feel safe. I'm on the lookout for nasty people.	0	1	2	3	4			
6	I worry a lot about the well-being of family and/or whether my professionals like me or not.	0	1	2	3	4			
7	I suppose my parents did the best they could with what they had.	4	3	2	1	0			
8	My parents were wonderful, and my childhood was happy. These questions are annoying.	0	1	2	3	4			
9	I don't resent the people who brought me up. They weren't perfect, but did their best.	4	3	2	1	0			
10	When I think about my past, I feel angry, confused, or frightened.	0	1	2	3	4			
11 optional	As a child, sometimes I ran away, hid, or just panicked and didn't know what to do.	0	1	2	3	4			
12	I can't remember my childhood very well, or anyone who could say what happened.	0	1	2	3	4			
13	I find it annoying or unfair when people say my childhood affected how I am now.	0	1	2	3	4			
14	I say sorry to people a lot and I worry that people I care about aren't very well.	0	1	2	3	4			
15	The love and care children get is important for their health.	4	3	2	1	0			
16	Telling my life story doesn't help anyone, and I find it a bit nosy.	0	1	2	3	4			

17	People have said that I'm 'aggressive', 'passive-aggressive', or 'manipulative'.	0	1	2	3	4		
18	How I was brought up isn't important, and it's irritating to be asked about it.	0	1	2	3	4		
19	I want to talk about my childhood, but when I do, the memories are very painful.	0	1	2	3	4		
20	I am really thankful to the people I love because they helped me cope with my difficulties.	4	3	2	1	0		
OFFICE USE ONLY	Total HI							
	Total IP							
	Total FP							

Scoring and Interpreting the sQuERRS©

The QuERRS-2 is a rating scale that highlights features of early attachment relationships that will be expressed in relationships between clients and psychologists, physicians, social workers, counsellors and other professions who may offer psychological help. The scale has been developed with people from the UK, who have mild to moderate intellectual disabilities, due to a lack of measures of emotional attachment specifically designed for them. However, it may be useful for other groups. Professionals should have some working knowledge of attachment theory. The scale may be unsuitable for brief helping interventions where early experiences are not discussed (e.g. attending mindfulness courses, brief group interventions for depression, etc). In clinical use, practitioners should present results to clients tactfully and to reflect the positive and adaptive elements of their attachment representational and behavioural systems i.e. how these strategies were effective ways of managing emotions and relationships in the past. For example, initially, it may be helpful to explain heightened independence less in terms of its avoidant elements, and to acknowledge the achievement in merely engaging with the therapy conversation, when one's model of relationships includes the expectation of being hurt or rebuffed.

The QuERRS-2 produces three scores:

■ Heightened independence (HI) refers to a general unwillingness to link past relationship experiences with current emotional functioning. HI may map on to dismissing attachment in adults (avoidant attachment in children). For those with high HI scores, therapy may be perceived as irritating or intrusive, or simply of little value, and there may be difficulties with engagement. Where a therapeutic encounter can be achieved, it may be difficult to construct a clear, factual personal story in formulation. Low or very low HI scores, by contrast, will be associated with ease in recalling the past, and whether positive or negative, and life experiences will be remembered realistically. Low HI scores are associated with lower clinical severity on presentation for help. Clinicians may find such individuals relatively easy to connect with, and help received is more likely to be welcomed and acted upon. Low HI may indicate autonomous attachment in adults (corresponding to secure attachment in children).

■ Interpersonal pain (IP) refers to current feelings of high distress that are commonly (but not exclusively) related to past neglect or maltreatment, and current interpersonal conflict. High IP scores are associated with more therapeutic session requirements, and higher severity of symptoms at presentation. Depending on engagement, this pain may be amenable to therapeutic intervention, although improvements in relationship functioning may be required before the person feels better internally. High IP may map on to unresolved attachment (disorganisation attachment in children) with a breakdown of coherent strategies for dealing with stressful encounters.

■ Fearful preoccupation (FP) refers to ongoing difficulties in feeling safe within current relationships. A positive aspect of high FP scores is that they are associated with greater gains in therapy (which should be a safe encounter). Higher scores may imply a preoccupation with the well-being of a significant other, or even the therapist, on whom some temporary dependency may be required prior to functioning independently. FP may map on to preoccupied attachment in adults (ambivalent attachment in children). Some people, especially those with mild or moderate intellectual difficulties, may need to develop permanent arrangements for physical and emotional safety, prior to exploratory work in therapy.

Suggested categorisation system for QuERRS-2 scores			
Scale score	Low	Intermediate	Elevated
Heightened independence	<10	10-31	>31
Interpersonal pain	<5	5-13	>13
Fearful preoccupation	<3	3-8	>8

Chapter 7:
Trauma-informed care in a service-related context

Elisabeth Goad

This book has already explored the significant levels of relational trauma experienced by people with intellectual disabilities in comparison to those in the general population (see also Jones *et al.,* 2012; Leeb *et al.,* 2012). The book has also touched on the conceptualisation of psychological trauma represented both in the form of the diagnosis post-traumatic stress disorder, but also in the sense of a process that can happen within relationships. Existing as a social experience, as well as an individual one, the realms of how psychological trauma is understood within intellectual disability (ID) services is finally progressing. Across all kinds of trauma lies a heightened sense of threat to reminders of the experience itself. With relational trauma, relationships themselves are the perceived threat often leading to interpersonal relationships feeling threatening in the person's current life as a result.

However, regardless of whether trauma occurs within relationships or not, its antidote is certainly within relationships. One human process by which to address this is through the flow of compassion (Gilbert, 2014). Compassion is a word often synonymous with health services (for example, compassionate leadership agendas, West, 2017; and being a common part of NHS core values) due to its positive impact on health care. Where organisations mirror their staff's core values of compassion, staff motivation and creativity are sustained, as well as higher levels of patient satisfaction and better health outcomes (West, 2017).

Compassion is intrinsically linked with the affiliative emotion regulation system written widely about by Paul Gilbert (e.g. Gilbert, 2014). The development of this system is impacted by early attachment experiences. Where there are attachment-related difficulties early in life, it can become under-developed (Mikulincer & Shaver, 2007). An under-developed affiliative emotional regulation system may leave the person under-resourced in regulating the threat processes commonly heightened with relational trauma. This can make it more difficult to feel connected and safe within themselves and, importantly, with others (Gilbert, 2009). However, strengthening the affiliative system has been evidenced to regulate the highly sensitive threat system in neurobiological studies (Gilbert, 2017). Doing so helps to address trauma-related distress (Lee, 2012). Those who have experienced relational trauma may feel most threatened within relationships. This may be especially true for those associated with power imbalance, such as between healthcare provider and service user. As such, our own relationships with service users and the relationships they have with our teams and organisations have the ability to either be re-traumatising, through replaying previous negative patterns of relating, or to become reparative experiences through the opportunity to experience caring relationships positively. Finding ways to ensure that every interaction (with us or our organisation) is an intervention (Treisman, 2017) is one basis of trauma-informed care.

However, a service-wide approach to trauma-informed care is complicated because of the complex interplay between professionals, service users and the organisation. This chapter focuses on the ideas underpinning the development (ever evolving) of one approach to trauma-informed care in community ID services in Surrey. It considers key initial steps in integrating this framework within healthcare services based upon the work developing within our own NHS trust.

What are the blocks to trauma-informed care (TIC)?

On an individual level there are many blocks to trauma-informed care. This can include how our own attachment behavioural systems can (and do) interact with those of our colleagues and service users (Marmarosh *et al.,* 2014) pulling us into all sorts of less-than-helpful relational loops. Additionally, sitting with the suffering of others can be very difficult indeed. It can often feel easier to minimise, avoid or oppress the difficult feelings associated with facing distress (Ballatt and Campling, 2011). Furthermore, health staff are often confronted with the idea that they may not be equipped to meet profound need, leading to feelings that may include compassion, but also may include anger and hostility too (Ballatt and Campling, 2011).

Organisational challenges are also no secret in healthcare services. Within teams, staff are often conflicted in their values on what they can see a person needs and the fit with the resource and capacity of the organisation. The Mid-Staffordshire NHS scandal (Francis, 2010) is just one example of how external threats (for example, huge financial deficits and punitive target-driven cultures) can, in turn, overwrite compassion with a threat-filled culture. Threat-filled cultures will impact on healthcare staff by influencing how they understand, respond and contribute to the organisational culture.

Though normal for the circumstance, these responses should be understood in order to protect against them undermining the interpersonal process between healthcare staff and service users. Organisations who can recognise the inter-relationship between these human based systems are those who have the ability to provide trauma-informed care through the context of a safe and connected organisation.

The questions below may help reflect upon these issues in the context of a healthcare organisation:

1. What do we need to do and, importantly, how do we need to be in order to help service users feel safe, contained and cared for enough to help regulate their threat systems?
2. What awareness do we have of what raises our own and our organisation's threat systems?
3. How do threat systems influence our interactions to be reparative, or re-traumatising?

Getting started, setting up TIC in a service context: starting conversations and gaining support

Feeling safe is paramount to human existence (Keesler, 2014). Where physical, emotional and social safety has been compromised, rebuilding social safety and connectedness with others is particularly important. If trauma-informed services aim to enable the people who use our services to feel safe within our care, then staff members also need to feel relationally safe in order to provide reparative care experiences. As the connection between service users and the organisation, staff require their own social safeness alongside connection with their own values and the values promoted (overtly and covertly) by the organisation itself.

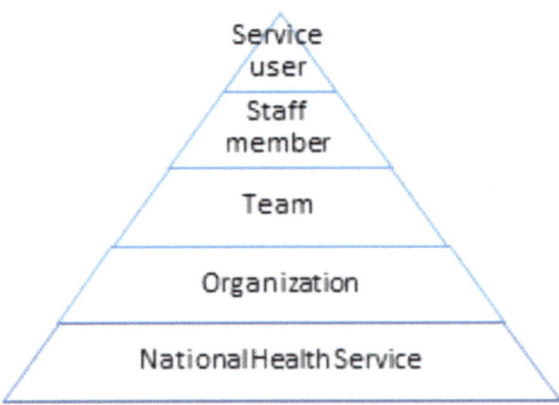

Figure 7.1: Hierarchy of safeness triangle

Figure 7.1 illustrates the multiple layers needed to help service users to experience services as safe and containing. Each layer can be understood as the solid foundation needed to stabilise the layer above to facilitate service users experiencing services as trauma-informed.

To develop a culture shift whereby the values of trauma-informed care are prioritised by staff and organisations, one needs to understand the organisation's readiness for change. Staff will also need to have an understanding about what it might mean for their own roles (Trauma-Informed Oregon, 2017). Although some have suggested that new initiatives should start from the top (e.g. Handran, 2013), others suggest that top-down initiatives are not the way to develop sustained change (West *et al.*, 2014). A careful distinction needs to be made here. Initiatives started from the 'top' generally do not yield success where staff feel 'done to' rather than 'done with'. However, in order to be successful, all initiatives must have support from the top of the organisation to help reduce potential barriers and to be enabled to grow. Considering how such support might be obtained as early as possible is a precursor for long-term success.

The blocks to trauma-informed care were discussed earlier in this chapter because understanding what organisational blocks are is an important starting point. Understanding the interrelationship between blocks and the impact on change can progress (NIHCE, 2007) should not be underestimated as the building blocks for solid foundations moving forward.

Figure 7.2 shares a set of key questions to facilitate reflection about blocks, barriers and readiness to change at the individual, team and organisational level.

-What is the team's current understanding of TIC?

-How closely are staff members' own professional models aligned with a TIC model of understanding human distress?

-What are our staff members' own key values and how does TIC support that?

-How can ways to engage people be found and pockets of enthusiasm utilized to realize the possibilities TIC presents within services?

-What were the key barriers to change on an individual, team and organizational level?

-Who might need to support the work, in what way and at what point?

-What impact do staff need to see on their clinical work? What actions are required for which outcomes in order for staff to see TIC as worth investing in to.

-How might TIC become part of the agenda across different staff groups (i.e. frontline,

---

Figure 7.2: Assessing the readiness of a frontline clinical team for embracing TIC (Goad, in press)

Conversations with whom?

Some teams and organisations will be more familiar with the ideas and values of trauma-informed care than others. Building exposure through the language of the framework (i.e. 'what has happened to you?', not 'what is wrong with you?': NES, 2017) can take time. Consider:

1. How to begin building the TIC picture by thinking creatively about ways to bring ideas about TIC into everyday conversations in a non-threatening way. The systemic concept about the difference that makes the difference but is not too different (Bateson, 1971) can be helpful in introducing ideas in a way people are able to hear.

2. What kind of conversations are needed? Are gentle, curious and informal conversations with colleagues needed first? Or is the team ready for more formal sharing of ideas?

3. Are there opportunities to share ideas through presentations or experiential exercises at team or organisation level?

4. Can a trauma-informed perspective be offered at meetings/team formulation or consultation?

5. How can service user and carer perspectives be gained in safe but in non-tokenistic ways?

The importance of these conversations rather lies in the ability of the leader to notice and confront the unconscious processes at work within teams when confronted with change. Bion (1968) has described the 'fight and flight' of the basic assumption principle in his group theory as a response to a problem that is either attacked or fled from. This is often as a defence in order to manage the often-conflicted feelings the problem might evoke. For example, the introduction of TIC may be seen as attacking and critical, should it provoke feelings of guilt about what should have been obvious (e.g. Winterbourne View, Whorlton Hall), leading often to avoidance of its reality and a rejection of those who raise such external reality (Stokes, 1994). Carefully negotiated conversations balancing the conscious needs of the team with the unconscious processes that can often otherwise undermine positive change are crucial. There are many theories and models that can underpin TIC and careful consideration of which is most appropriate to enable the team to connect with it is crucial early decision.

The concept of psychological trauma had been described by Freud following on from the First World War where he described the experiences of soldiers with what he termed traumatic neurosis, where a protective shield against overwhelming experiences breaks down, and the mind is flooded and bound to terror. To Freud (e.g. in *Beyond the Pleasure Principle*, 1920) this reflected internal conflict within the individual's fantasy life rather than being a relational phenomenon (West, 2016). However, Freud suggests that real-world trauma can have a significant impact on one's attachments as trauma indicates 'what life would be like with no attachments at all'.

Later, although under-acknowledged until the advent of relational approaches, Bowlby (1980) focused on real-world trauma and its relational impact with his attachment theory, which also remains an important part of current thinking. More recently, compassion-focused therapy (Gilbert, 2014) and systemic theory (see James and MacKinnon, 2012) have further expanded upon relational conceptualisation of traumatic experiences. Choosing a theoretical underpinning, within which to situate TIC, will ensure that the framework can be reality-tested. However, in some ways, it may matter less about which theory or associated the practitioner prefers, than which is most accessible to the most people. In the context of engaging care staff in conversations about trauma (many of whom will not have training in psychological theory about trauma), a model should be chosen that is relatively easy to understand. If there are models used already within the team that are compatible with TIC, could these be built upon. If there are pockets of helpful language within the team, these people may be able to help advocate for the framework as they may naturally be more closely aligned.

Consider staff well-being

Staff well-being is a significant part of TIC. The evidence that caring for staff is the key to providing compassionate care is now overwhelmingly strong (See West *et al.,* 2017). The sooner staff well-being is prioritised, the more likely staff are to feel that TIC is worth investing their energy in to. To start with, this might just be thinking about the basics, such as environmental safety, training opportunities and the ability to take all of their annual leave rather than concerning ourselves with coffee machines and conference freebies. Find time to ask genuinely about:

1. What do staff feel they need from each other?
2. What do staff feel they need from their managers?
3. What do staff feel they need from their organisation?
4. How do we reach a level of resilience that allows us to work effectively?

The outcomes of these discussions are of course then subject to negotiating conversations about what can be achieved. However, focusing on what can be done on the key themes raised can help creatively increase morale and staff support.

Building the identity of TIC

One early dilemma to consider is how TIC fits with the identity of the organisation. This refers to its culture but also, more specifically, to the other policies and agendas that are prioritised.

1. How does TIC 'fit'? How is it the same as other initiatives?
2. How is it different from other initiatives?

An initiative too similar may be seen as unworthy of additional time and resource. One that is too different, may threaten or undermine other agendas. An organisational tightrope must be walked. Examples of where TIC aligns strongly with current priorities include Transforming Care (DoH, 2012) after the horrendous abuse uncovered at Winterbourne View. It aligns with the 'positive and safe' agenda (DoH, 2014) in concerning itself with reducing restraint and a variety of well-being initiatives as staff well-being is as important a part of its remit as service user experience because the two are so intrinsically linked.

However, there are differences too. Historically, many policies and agendas have laid out a series of objectives to be achieved in order to improve care. Yet it is not uncommon to see that, despite clear steps set out in well-intended policy, they have not always been achieved. An example of this may lie in Transforming Care (2014) where Taylor *et al.* (2017; Taylor, 2019) question its evidence base, its underlying assumptions and its inability to better equip community services to cope with a decrease in inpatient beds. However, in this and many other policies, one area with less focus are interpersonal processes; between ourselves but also within the systems within which we reside, and how these might, at times, undermine achieving the objectives set out before us. What makes TIC different is that it is the link that pulls all other agendas together; the umbrella framework that interweaves with all other policies. It guides not only the content of what is done but also guides the 'how' in terms of the interpersonal processes required to provide consistently compassionate care.

Understanding and articulating the identity of TIC in relation to other agendas will help to navigate its progress in an often-complex organisational context. Figure 7.3 highlights considerations in exploring trauma-informed identity in the context of the wider organisation.

> -*What are the important agendas and priorities within the team and organization?*
> -*Do these agendas align or clash with trauma-informed care?*
> -*How might differences and similarities be managed?*
> -*What are the core values underpinning individual, team and organizational identity and how does this fit with trauma-informed care?*

Figure 7.3: Trauma-informed identity (Goad, in press)

Winterbourne View and Whorlton Hall were saying the right things. They had words like 'compassion' all over the walls. Yet, was care good enough? No. We know we need to do something differently but people are very anxious about change so need to prove its worth – help people understand this.

Finding a way to offer all staff a voice: Increasing knowledge, addressing power differentials and enabling all staff to have a voice

It has already been understood that relational processes are a key component of TIC. There are complex and interlinked relationships between our clients, ourselves and our organisations. Yet, historically, health services have taken rather a dichotomous approach between 'us' providing treatment and 'them' receiving it. Richards *et al.* (2016) talk extensively about the service user/professional identity split. The idea that service users are somehow different can at times keep us removed from their (and our) experiences as fellow human beings. This may be a defence against work that at times feels emotionally challenging, but it does not help develop the openness needed to engage with ideas about our interpersonal interactions being as important as the content of any intervention offered. Within ID services, we have the fortitude of multiple professional groups within teams. However, not all will have trained with a focus on interpersonal process. Where there are different professional groups, there are also power hierarchies that make it more difficult for some staff to have their voices heard comparatively to others. These differences may relate to years of experience, qualification, status of the profession and other social graces such as gender, race, class, and level of education (Burnham, 2012). TIC values all people as equal, and all types of staff knowledge and experience as important. Thus, finding a way to hear all voices is a priority.

There are many different ways to enable voices within the team. Offering introductory training and a reflective space early on may help the team develop a shared language from which to speak and to bring everyone on to a more level playing field. Reflective practice is well evidenced to positively enable better quality of care (e.g. Hoge, Migdole, Cannata and Powell, 2014). Whether in reflective practice groups or within supervision, it provides two important functions within TIC. Firstly, by adopting a trauma-informed lens to reflect from within, it may prevent the re-traumatisation of clients due to clinician or organisational processes that might otherwise be held out of conscious awareness. Secondly, by acknowledging vicarious traumatisation of staff through continually 'bearing witness' to the trauma narratives told to them but also due to the system they work within. For example, trauma has been systemically linked to homophobia, racism, sexism, classism and ethnoreligious oppression (Quiros and Berger, 2015). Reflective space to understand both power and privilege within staff members often enables stronger working alliances in the context of a more helpful focus on clients (Phillips *et al.,* 2016). Training is also an important step initially as facilitating change can be difficult if staff feel they do not have the confidence and knowledge to work in a trauma-informed way (Isobel and Edwards, 2017).

Figure 7.4 below summarises the main training objectives for the introductory training sessions run in Surrey ID services.

- Building the context around TIC and how it fits with our values as healthcare professionals
- Sharing strengths as a staff team and staying psychologically safe
- Understanding what trauma means in the context of TIC
- Understanding diagnosis in the context of TIC
- The basics of attachment theory situated in the theory of compassion
- Three emotional regulation systems: how they help understand how we feel and respond to others
- Relational trauma: how it fits with attachment
- Neuro-sequential understanding of trauma (Perry & Dobson, 2013)
- Re-traumatizing healthcare
- Trauma and diversity
- Trauma-Informed Care: What actually is it?
- Trauma-Informed Care and attachment

Figure 7.4: Potential training objectives for TIC (Goad, in press)

However, it has long been known that training alone is not enough to develop and maintain new ways of working (Torrey *et al.*, 2012). As such, a significant proportion of the session was a reflective space for staff to consider what was important to them about the kind of care they wanted to provide and what might block achieving this. From this, a set of priorities were developed. A blend of 'quick wins' to maintain motivation versus longer-terms goals was a good balance. Objectives were clearly defined with clear action points and staff teams were involved in prioritising actions to start with change that felt meaningful to them.

Picking a small set of actions to develop first, utilising different working groups for each one, help professionals feel more able to sign up rather than feeling overwhelmed by the magnitude of the task in hand. Building confidence in the multidisciplinary team (MDT) that everyone has something to offer is paramount to all members of the MDT being central to this approach (Truesdale *et al.*, 2019). TIC is a human process. In its simplest form, it is a transactional process rather than an academic or clinical one. Having the confidence within all members of the MDT is crucial for its success.

Pre and post training questionnaires completed across both community teams suggested that staff members:

Felt more confident in:

- Recognising different attachment patterns and how different attachment patterns might impact people using services.
- Asking people about whether they have experienced psychological trauma.
- responding helpfully to someone disclosing a traumatic experience
  Their ability to understand their own life experiences in interaction with your clients.

A thematic analysis of the semi-structured interviews completed with staff who had attended the training draw themes summarised as the following:

- Staff felt their knowledge and confidence had increased about trauma-informed care, also demonstrated through their use of language.
- Staff were able to draw links from the training to their clinical practice.
- Staff found the training emotionally evocative but valued this as important.
- Staff valued the training as inclusive in bringing all professions together.
- Staff talked of barriers to implementation.
- Staff valued the way the training modelled trauma-informed care with its set up focused on staff wellbeing.

Figure 7.5: Training outcomes for the ID division at SABP (Goad, in press)

Developing a framework or model for change

Where staff have a few clearly defined objectives, they are more innovative and provide better care than teams without such clarity (West *et al.*, 2014). As such, providing a visual representation of the main objectives that have been agreed by the team can be helpful in maintaining focus and sharing direction with management across the organisation. Others are more likely to support the process if they can better understand the direction of travel. The clearer and better defined the objectives are, the easier it is to develop a set of specific actions with associated outcome measures.

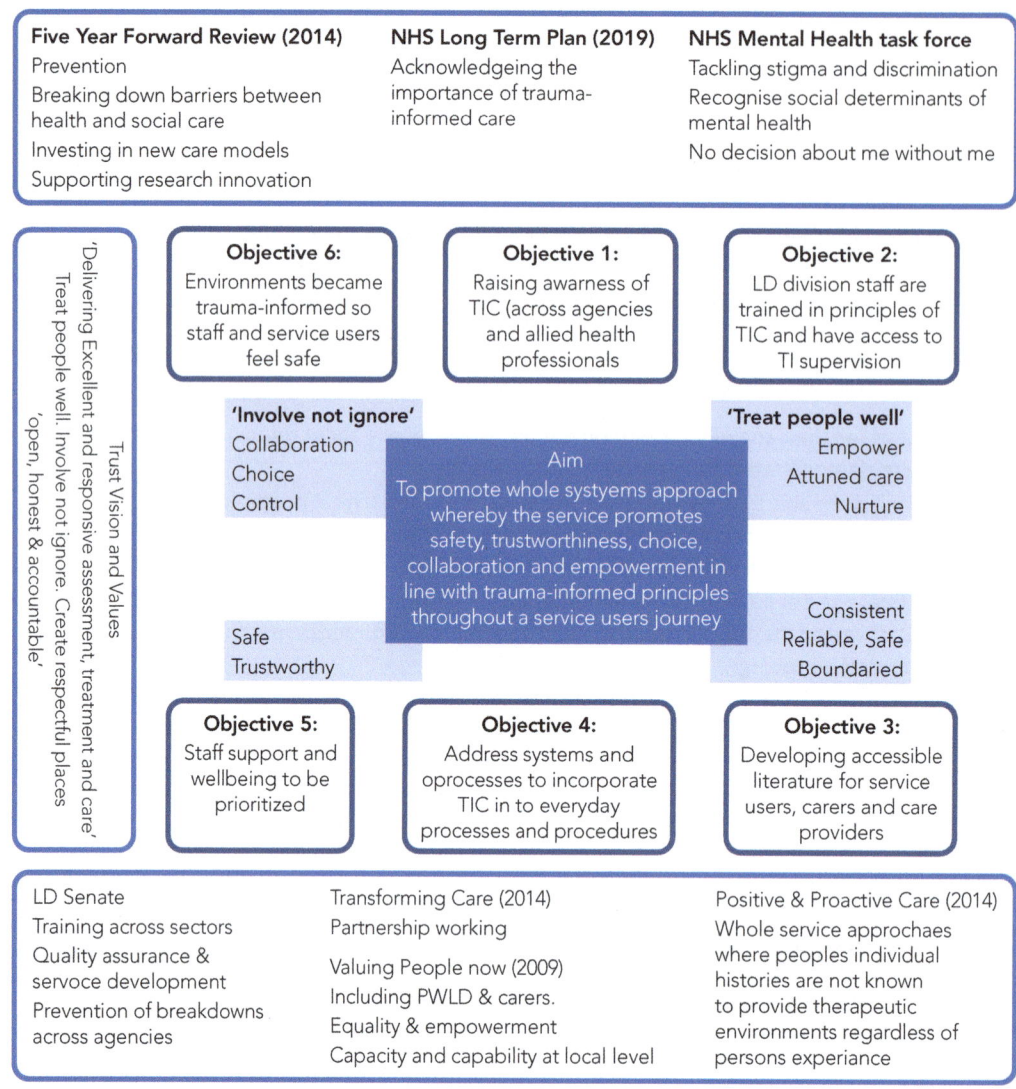

Five Year Forward Review (2014)
Prevention
Breaking down barriers between health and social care
Investing in new care models
Supporting research innovation

NHS Long Term Plan (2019)
Acknowledgeing the importance of trauma-informed care

NHS Mental Health task force
Tackling stigma and discrimination
Recognise social determinants of mental health
No decision about me without me

'Delivering Excellent and responsive assessment, treatment and care'
Treat people well. Involve not ignore. Create respectful places
'open, honest & accountable'

Trust Vision and Values

Objective 6:
Environments became trauma-informed so staff and service users feel safe

Objective 1:
Raising awarness of TIC (across agencies and allied health professionals

Objective 2:
LD division staff are trained in principles of TIC and have access to TI supervision

'Involve not ignore'
Collaboration
Choice
Control

Aim
To promote whole systyems approach whereby the service promotes safety, trustworthiness, choice, collaboration and empowerment in line with trauma-informed principles throughout a service users journey

'Treat people well'
Empower
Attuned care
Nurture

Consistent
Reliable, Safe
Boundaried

Safe
Trustworthy

Objective 5:
Staff support and wellbeing to be prioritized

Objective 4:
Address systems and oprocesses to incorporate TIC in to everyday processes and procedures

Objective 3:
Developing accessible literature for service users, carers and care providers

LD Senate
Training across sectors
Quality assurance & servoce development
Prevention of breakdowns across agencies

Transforming Care (2014)
Partnership working
Valuing People now (2009)
Including PWLD & carers.
Equality & empowerment
Capacity and capability at local level

Positive & Proactive Care (2014)
Whole service approchaes where peoples individual histories are not known to provide therapeutic environments regardless of persons experiance

Figure 7.6: Provisional visionary model developed with staff within Surrey community ID teams (Goad, in press)

Figure 7.6 illustrates one visual representation focusing on a clear aim and set of basic objectives for the team, situated within both LD-specific and NHS agendas. The model presents only a dynamic starting point. As new people, and thus ideas, enter the conversation about TIC, it will evolve into richer territories. It should not be viewed as a static entity. Although it is not within the scope of this chapter to break down the detail of each objective; figure 7.7 illustrates examples of the more tangible elements within a sample of objectives.

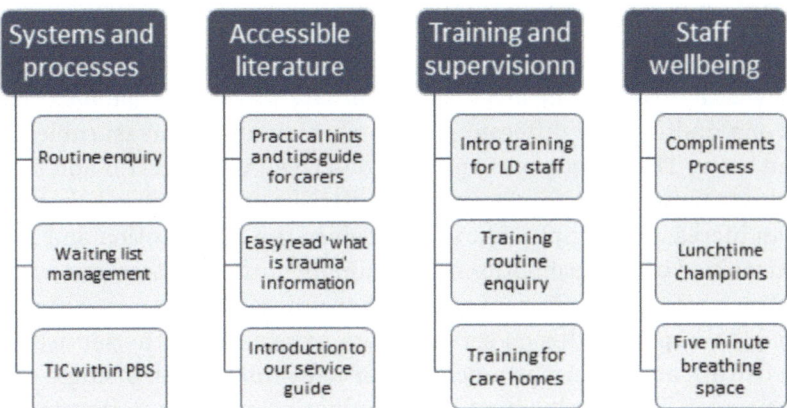

Figure 7.7: Examples of objectives broken down in to a sample of their specific areas for action

Figure 7.7 is a brief snapshot rather than an exhaustive list. Its intention is to help illustrate examples of TIC in practice and to bring what can feel like an abstract concept into more tangible and achievable goals. To take this one step further, figure 7.8 below illustrates a brief summary of the process and outcomes of one of the most tangible elements focusing on re-developing team compliment processes.

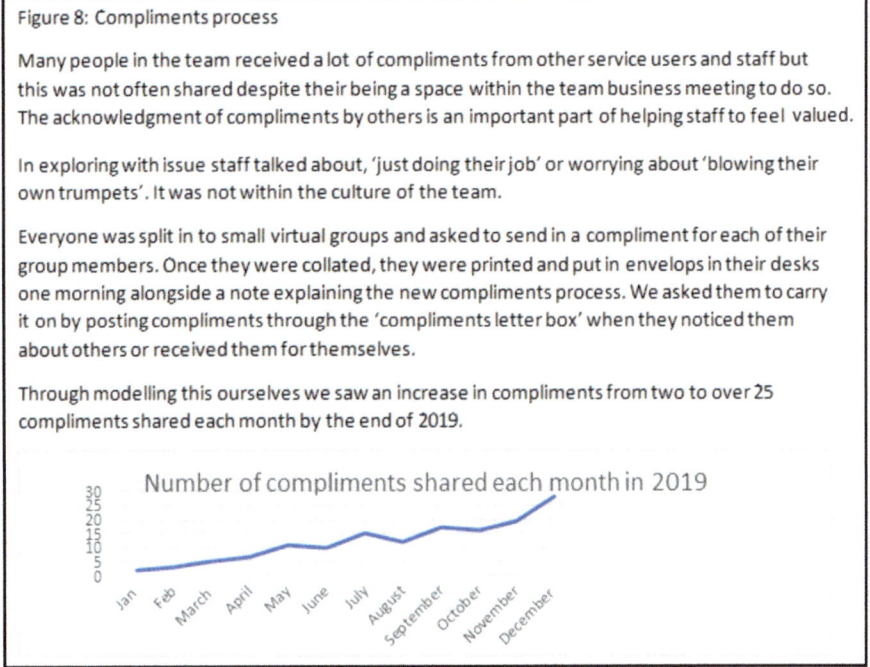

Figure 7.8: Compliments process

A word about evaluation

The subject of evaluation deserves a chapter on its own but the most important thing to say is that there is no one way to evaluate TIC. It is a complex construct composed of a multitude of different elements which are all measurable; but in different ways. The compliments process described in figure 7.8 and the introductory training sessions are simpler initiatives to measure. It is easy to measure an increase in compliment sharing since the intervention and see whether this is maintained over the months, or to evaluate staff members' knowledge and confidence before and after introductory training. However, it is harder to understand the impact of this on service users' experience of the service. TIC is a change in culture and culture is much harder to evaluate than a single concrete change in process. The development of an evaluation strategy in its own right might be a helpful place to start. Considerations include:

- evaluation as a web of measures rather than a singular one. There is no one way to measure the success of TIC.

- service evaluation and audits form an important part of evaluation and are often a quick, manageable way to understanding change in fast-moving clinical environments.

- a combination of quantitative and qualitative measures to help develop a richer understanding of both concrete change, and staff and service-user experience.

- if organisations use a quality improvement framework, this can be incorporated into the evaluation strategy.

- evaluation could include a range of different perspectives including staff, service user and carers.

- Evaluation could include analysis of concrete changes in process and outcome (i.e. effectiveness of training) as well as culture change indicators (i.e. analysis of staff language).

The importance of defining outcome measures that can measure all elements of systemic change lies in both working towards positive change for service users and carers but also to motivate staff by illustrating that TIC is clinically helpful. Outcomes might seek to evaluate knowledge and confidence of staff (from training), changes in behaviour (increase in sharing compliments), monitoring staff sickness, understanding the impact of attachment (particularly avoidant, preoccupied and disorganised patterns) on clinical outcomes, understanding the impact of adversity in mental health outcomes, number of restraints on inpatient wards, and so on. It might also evaluate the introduction of support systems for staff to reprocess difficult experiences leading to vicarious traumatisation or pathways to specialist support in trauma-focused psychotherapies for people who use our services. More broadly of course, one might hope to bear witness to a reduction in the catastrophic and deeply traumatising events at Winterborne View, Whorlton Hall and similar scandals, rather than engaging in avoidance.

A final note

This chapter has shared ideas about the practical application of TIC within a healthcare context. There will be several approaches to this, and thus its intention is to stimulate the thinking needed to begin relating some of the ideas to the reader's own area of clinical practice, rather than offer a more directive step-by-step guide. It is based on the experiences of developing TIC within the ID division in Surrey and Borders Partnership NHS Foundation Trust. However, it is important to note that we see ourselves as 'taking steps towards' rather than 'being' trauma-informed. This approach enables us to maintain our curiosity on how our processes fit (or do not fit) with the framework of TIC as the conversation continues.

As always, healthcare staff are our biggest asset. Taking the time to find out and utilise different staff members' unique strengths and qualities help drive forward progress. TIC might feel like a large task in today's cash-strapped health services, but the most important thing is to just start somewhere. Tackling one process or making one change can all start changing a culture to one privileging the key question of 'what happened to you rather than what is wrong with you,' (NES, 2017), which as we know is the crux of TIC.

A worked example of trauma-informed care in a community intellectual disability team

Callum was a young 25 year old man who loved 'films based on a true story', running (a lot) and going for long walks. e also had a diagnosis of a moderate intellectual disability, AD D and autism. Callum was referred to the community team for people with intellectual disabilities following on a placement breakdown which had led to him moving in to our geographical area.

Callum's referral letter stated that he presented with several behaviours that challenged including verbal and physical aggression, obsessions over certain staff members and refusal to work with others. The referral information suggested that Callum had experienced multiple placement breakdowns including as a child when he was taken in and out of care as his parents struggled to cope.

Callum was Invited for initial assessment wherebyhis whole health needs were assessed. From there it was agreed with Callum and his carers to attend a joint psychology and psychiatry appointment. Although there was a waiting list for psychology, the initial appointment was completed quickly so that a fuller picture could be developed, initial advice and support offered and any other appropriate referrals identified and made. Routine enquiry during these initial meetings was considered and based on concerns about Callum's receptive communication, high anxiety levels in the appointment and voiced uncertainty from care staff about how to support him, it didn't feel a safe enough environment to ask Callum specifically about his past relational experiences. As such, the question was asked, 'is there anything else about your life that you think is important to tell me?'. This modelled an openness to hearing his story that might enable him to tell us what he felt we needed to know as he built more trust in us. The initial appointment process was supported by easy read materials by our team about what we do and what would happen next.

With permission, previous notes were sought and communication with other professionals was made in order to ensure that Callum's care was joined up and that all relevant information was shared to inform his current care. Referrals were also made to Occupational Therapy in relation to Callum's sensory needs and Speech and language Therapy due to his communication needs. Due to waiting, lists within the service, not all professionals were able to pick up Callum's case straight away. Given his history of neglect, we were concerned about how we might ensure Callum waiting for support did not re-trigger experiences of being abandoned. As such, we offered regular check in calls to ensure that Callum knew he was being held in mind and also to offer further advice/support prior to full support being offered.

As part of the intervention, we worked with all parts of the system where possible. We focused initially on developing a provisional trauma-informed formulation to enable the development of a positive behavioural support plan based heavily on attachment principles. A real emphasis was placed on offering staff support and thinking with managers about developing a supportive environment for staff where problems could be discussed safely without blame and regular communication avenues and supervision structures were developed. Trauma-informed training focused on developing awareness of unconscious interpersonal processes, highlighting the importance of the interpersonal nature of the work alongside offering space for thoughts and feelings to be reflected upon in a safe environment. Understanding the strengths of both Callum and the support team were paramount throughout and used towards the end of the work as to how they might further build on their successes together in the future. The ending of the work was celebrated and therapeutic letters and social stories written highlighting all that had been valued about both Callum and the staff team. At the end of the work there had been no incidents of aggression for 16 weeks, Callum had stable relationships with group of 6-8 staff who supported him regularly and the staff had been able to turn their focus from behaviours that challenge to supporting Callum to focus on his own identity and the important elements of his life that he wanted to rediscover.

Figure 7.9: A worked example of trauma-informed care in a community intellectual disability team

References

Ballatt J & Campling P (2011) *Intelligent Kindness. Reforming the culture of healthcare* (1st Edition). London: The Royal College of Psychiatrists.

Bateson G (1971) A Re-examination of 'Bateson's Rule'. *Journal of Genetics* **60** 230–240.

Bion WR (1968) *Experiences in Groups*: London: Tavistock Publications.

Bowlby J (1980) *Attachment and Loss, volume 111: Loss, sadness and depression*. London, UK: The Hogarth Press and the Institute of Psycho-Analysis.

Burnham J (2012) Developments in social GRRAAACCEEESSS: Visible-invisible and voiced-unvoiced. In: IB Krouse (Eds) *Culture and Reflexivity in Systemic Psychotherapy: Mutual perspectives* (pp139-160). London and New York: Karnac books Ltd.Department of Health (2009) Valuing People Now: A new three-year strategy for learning disabilities. London: Department of Health.

Department of Health (2012) *Transforming Care: A National response to Winterbourne View hospital*. London: Department of Health.

Department of Health (2014) *Positive and proactive care: Reducing the need for restrictive interventions* [online]. London: Department of Health: Available at: assets.publishing.service.gov.uk

Francis R (2010) *The Independent Inquiry into Care Provided by Mid-Staffordshire NHS Foundation Trust, January 2005-March 2009* [online]. London: HMSO. Available from: https://assets.publishing.service.gov.uk/government/uploads/system/uploads/attachment_data/file/279109/0375_i.pdf

Freud S (1920/2003) Beyond the Pleasure Principle. In A Phillips (ed) *Beyond the Please Principle and Other Writings* (1st edition) (pp45–102). New York: Penguin Books.

Gilbert P (2009) *The Compassionate Mind*. London: Constable & Robinson.

Gilbert P (2014) The origins and nature of compassion focused therapy. *British Journal of Clinical Psychology* **53** (1) 6–41.

Gilbert P (2017) *Compassion. Concepts, Research and Applications*. London and New York: Routledge.

Goad E (in press) Working alongside people with intellectual disabilities who have had difficult experiences: Reflections on trauma-informed care within a service context. *Journal of Intellectual Disabilities*

Handran J (2013) *Trauma-informed organisational culture: The prevention, reduction, and treatment of compassion fatigue*. Thesis. Colorado State University. Available at: https://mountainscholar.org/bitstream/handle/10217/78825/Handran_colostate_0053A_11673.pdf.

Hoge MA, Migdole S, Cannata E, & Powell D (2014). Strengthening supervision in systems of care: Exemplary practices in empirically supported treatments. *Clinical Social Work Journal* **42** (2), 171–181.

Isobel S & Edwards C (2017) Using trauma informed care as a nursing model of care in an acute inpatient mental health unit: A practice development process. *International Journal of Mental Health Nursing* **26** (1) 88–94.

James K & MacKinnon L (2012) Integrating a trauma lens into a family therapy framework: Ten principles for family therapists. *Australian and New Zealand Journal of Family Therapy, Special Issue on Family Therapy and Trauma* **33** (3) 189–209.

Jones L, Bellis MA, Wood S, Hughes K, McCoy E, Eckley L, Bates G (2012) Prevalence and risk of violence against adults with disabilities: A systematic review and meta-analysis of observational studies. *Lancet* **379** (9845) 1621–1629.

Keesler JM (2014) A call for the integration of trauma-informed care among intellectual and developmental disability organisations. *Journal of Policy and Practice in Intellectual Disabilities* **11** (1) 34–42.

Lee DA (2012) *The Compassionate Mind Approach to Recovering from Trauma*. London: Constable & Robinson.

Leeb RT, Bitsko RH, Merrick MT & Armour BS (2012) Does childhood disability increase risk for child abuse and neglect? *Journal of Mental Health Research in Intellectual Disabilities* **5** 4–31.

Marmarosh CL, Kivlighan DM, Bieri K, LaFauci Schutt JM, Barone C, Choi J (2014) The insecure psychotherapy base: Using client and therapist attachment styles to understand the early alliance. *Psychotherapy*, **51** (3) 404–412.

Marriot C, Parish C, Griffiths C & Fish R. (2019) Experiences of shame and intellectual disabilities: Two case studies. *Journal of Intellectual Disabilities, 1-14*. Available at: http://www.research.lancs.ac.uk/portal/en/publications/experiences-of-shame-and-intellectual-disabilities(3dc0e0e8-62bc-47c0-a8e8-fde7b8a4801a)/export.html.

Mikulincer M & Shaver PR (2007) *Attachment in Adulthood: Structure, dynamics, and change*. New York: Guildford Press.

National Institute for Health and Clinical Excellence (2007) *How to change practice. Understand, identify and overcome barriers to change*. London: National Institute for Health and Clinical Excellence.

National LD Professional Senate (2015) *Delivering Effective Specialist Community Learning Disabilities Health Team Support to People with Learning Disabilities and their Families or Carers*. LD Professional Senate.

NHS England (2014) *Five year forward view* [online]. Available at: https://www.england.nhs.uk/wp-content/uploads/2014/10/5yfv-web.pdf

NHS England (2019) *The NHS Long Term Plan* [online]. Available at: https://www.longtermplan.nhs.uk/wp-content/uploads/2019/08/nhs-long-term-plan-version-1.2.pdf

NHS Education for Scotland (2017). *Transforming psychological trauma: A knowledge and skills framework for the Scottish Workforce*. Edinburgh: Scottish Government Press.

Perry B & Dobson C (2013) The neurosequential model of therapeutics. In: J Ford and C Courtois (Eds) *Treating Complex Traumatic Stress Disorders in Children and Adolescents: Scientific foundations and therapeutic models* (PP 249-260). New York: Guilford Press.

Phillips JC, Parent MC, Dozier C, & Jackson PL (2016) Depth of discussion of multicultural identities in supervision and supervisory outcomes. *Counselling Psychology Quarterly* **30** (2) 188–210.

Quiros L & Berger R (2015). Responding to the sociopolitical complexity of trauma: An integration of theory and practice. *Loss and Trauma* **20** (2) 149–159.

Richards J, Holttum S & Springham, N (2016) How do 'mental health professionals' who are also or have been 'mental health service users' construct their identities? *SAGE Open* **6** (1) 1–14.

Stokes J (1994) Problems in multidisciplinary teams: The unconscious at work. *Journal of Social Work Practice* **8** (2) 161-167.

Taylor JL (2019) Delivering the Transforming Care Programme: A case of smoke and mirrors? *BJPsych Bulletin*, **43**, 201-203.

Taylor JL, McKinnon I, Thorpe I & Gillmer BT (2017) The impact of transforming care on the care and safety of patients with intellectual disabilities and forensic needs. *BJPsychBulletin*, **41**, 205-208.

The Transforming Care and Commissioning Group (2014) *Transforming Care: Time for Change. Transforming the commissioning of services for people with learning disabilities and / or autism* [online]. Available from: https://www.england.nhs.uk/wp-content/uploads/2014/11/transforming-commissioning-services.pdf.

Torrey W, Bond G, McHugo G & Swain K (2012) Evidence-based practice implementation in community mental health settings: The relative importance of key domains of implementation activity. *Administration and Policy of Mental Health* **39** (5) 353–364.

Trauma Informed Oregon (2017) *Creating Cultures Trauma Informed Care (CCTIC): A Self- Assessment and Planning Protocol*. Community Connections: Washington: Trauma Informed Oregon. Available at https://traumainformedoregon.org/wp-content/uploads/2014/10/CCTIC-A-Self-Assessment-and-Planning-Protocol.pdf

Treisman, K (2017) *Working with Relational and Developmental Trauma in Children and Adolescents*. Oxon and New York: Routledge.

Truesdale M, Brown, M, Taggart, L & Bradley, A (2019) Trauma-informed care: A qualitative study exploring the views and experiences of professionals in specialist health services for adults with intellectual disabilities. *Journal of Applied Research in Intellectual Disabilities* **32** (6) 1–9.

West MA, Topakas A, & Dawson JF (2014) Climate and culture for health care performance. In: B Schneider and KM Barbera (Eds) *The Oxford Handbook of Organisational Climate and Culture* (pp335–59). Oxford: Oxford University Press.

West M, Eckert R, Collins B & Chowla R (2017) *Caring to Change – How compassionate leadership can stimulate innovation in healthcare*. London: Kings Fund. Available from: https://www.kingsfund.org.uk/sites/default/files/field/field_publication_file/Caring_to_change_Kings_Fund_May_2017.pdf

Chapter 8: Providing emotionally aware care in the positive behavioural support framework

Cathy Harding

'Behaviours can be described as challenging when it is of such intensity, frequency or duration as to threaten the quality of life and / or the physical safety of the individual or others and is likely to lead to responses that are restrictive, adverse or result in exclusion.'
–Royal College of Psychiatry, British Psychological Society and Royal College of Speech and Language therapy, 2007. P 10

'There was no single moment, no magical epiphany, in which everything changed. Just as so much of the impact of trauma is death by a thousand paper cuts, I think so much of the benefit of therapy is in the drip-drip-drip; moments of feeling seen and feeling heard and feeling felt, moments of our nervous system starting to re-regulate back down into the green zone, and us slowly bringing our front brains back online.'
– Spring, 2018 podcast #2 Recovery is possible

An introduction to positive behavioural support and understanding complex developmental trauma within this framework

All behaviours have a meaning; and this is central to positive behaviour support (PBS). PBS is a broad approach combining tools of behavioural interventions and functional assessment with person-centred interventions including skill teaching, behavioural support plans, modelling, staff training, improving quality of life, enhancing community inclusion and integrating active support (Allan, 2009). Held central to this is to develop an understanding of the functions of these behaviours within the persons context.

PBS has emerged as a distinct approach to behavioural support due to its commitment to values and increasing quality of life for individuals (and their advocates) as defined by their personal choices (BILD *et al.,* 2017). This means that PBS aims to consider the person and his or her life circumstances, including physical health and emotional needs, such as the impact of any traumatic or adverse life events and mental illness (BILD *et al.,* 2017). As the quote from Spring (2020) highlights, there is no 'quick fix' in supporting individuals with trauma histories, but rather, individuals need to be supported over the longer-term. This is also the goal within PBS: a person-centred framework for providing long-term support. Furthermore, the relational experiences she talks about being needed can have a powerful impact when provided by care staff (and families) who support the person for their full day, extending the experience from just being within therapy.

PBS is a data-driven and values-based framework, which can incorporate a range of other psychological models such as trauma-informed care (TIC), autism-specific approaches, active support and other appropriate interventions that support physical, mental health and well-being (BILD, 2017). Whilst the evidence base is still growing, PBS is endorsed in policy and evidence and professional based guidance (e.g. RCP *et al.,* 2007; NICE, 2015). The behavioural theories underpinning PBS may seem at odds with the relational elements of trauma informed approaches, yet, PBS can be used to deliver support plans which incorporate trauma-informed ideas, in a way which enhances understanding and outcomes; especially when embedded within a trauma informed organisation.

This chapter aims to outline:

- how understanding trauma and trauma-related approaches can be embedded within a PBS framework

- how these approaches together can aid with understanding behaviours that challenge
- their development and function for individuals who have experienced trauma and the primary, secondary and reactive interventions which can aid with recovery.

It will look at how this understanding can be embedded within a PBS format, and allow staff to comprehensively support people who have had developmental trauma to develop secure and attuned relationships.

How trauma can look like behaviours that are challenging

In the *Practice Guidelines for Trauma Informed Care and Service Delivery* (Kezeler and Stravropoulos, 2012), it is discussed that the following behaviours are ways in which trauma might present in individuals: behaviours that are aggressive or violent; self-harm; refusal to co-operate or disobeying commands; withdrawal and sleeping at inappropriate times; hypersensitivity or sensation seeking; task and relationship avoidance; extreme attention seeking and/or poor social skills. Any of these could be a behaviour that challenges and therefore be responded to within a PBS framework.

There are other behaviours that these practice guidelines also record as common for individuals who have experienced trauma; these are recorded in Figure 8.1. These behaviours can offer further clues to trauma being the underlying cause of behaviours that challenge, and help to identify whether trauma may be a part of the function of behaviour. Intervening in these areas will aid with supporting trauma recovery and therefore shape primary preventative strategies within the PBS plan.

Figure 8.1: Behaviours associated with trauma	
From Kezeler and Stravropoulos, 2012	
■ Lying – weird explanations ■ Blaming others ■ 'Playing' people against each other ■ Focus on immediate and not wanting to talk about past ■ Unable to reflect on incidents ■ Compartmentalised memories ■ Disproportionate behaviour ■ Poor turn taking	■ Talking too much ■ Not understanding some words or dissociation ■ Misreading facile cues ■ Difficulties with proximity/touch ■ Preferring younger games ■ Chaos within life, not learning from mistakes ■ Hard to get to know/feel close to ■ Odd reactions and behaviours

How PBS fits alongside TIC

There are multiple elements to TIC, and this includes the importance of leadership, environments and culture. However, central to many models that focus on recovery from trauma, is the importance of a healing relationship, which is genuine and valuing (see Jackson and Waters, 2015). As emphasised in this quote by Spring (2020):

'We have experienced a wound; what we might call relational trauma. It's been perpetuated or caused by another human being. And we need to have reparative experience, an opposite experience, where instead of hurt and harm and abuse, we experience care and compassion and empathy. That has the potential to change the way we view other people, ourselves, and the nature of the world. It's very powerful.'
– Spring, 2019, podcast #7 Can we heal?

Within this genuine and valuing relationship, individuals can heal in multifaceted ways that are required following trauma, particularly complex trauma. The above quote by Spring (2020) provokes thought regarding the concept of relational security (Skelly, 2017). Within intellectual disability (ID) and trauma care, there is an emphasis on the importance of relational security and the provision of emotionally aware care; these elements fit neatly alongside the competencies within the positive behavioural support framework. The PBS competencies are values which we strive to meet when supporting individuals with behaviours that challenge, and include the service accomplishments of providing individuals with choice, being respectful, supporting community presence, participation and relationships (O`Brien, (1992). These competencies arguably enable or enhance a sense of relational security.

Relational security encompasses the elements of physical safety, emotional predictability, warmth, and shared joyful interactions and experiences (Skelly, 2016). The PBS plan can facilitate these elements of relational security. Relational security ensures that the individual is safe from physical harm, and in addition that they also feel as if they are safe. When we have numerous people with behaviours that challenge in the same places this may not be easily achieved. Absence of threat is an important element in physical safety, but it is not enough. There also needs to be the presence of connection where people feel seen, heard and accepted without judgement (Fowler, 2020). Also, consistency in emotional responses and allowing and valuing displays of warmth from staff is important. Shared, joyful interactions and experiences are an important element of relational security, but this can be particularly tricky with individuals with high levels of challenging behaviour, so having these experiences and ensuring that they are part of the narrative around an individual is important (e.g Coles and Ellis-Caird, 2019). These can be examined in part by the relational risk questions (Skelly, 2014). These questions aim to help examine whether there are relational elements that need to be considered alongside the functional assessment (see Figure 8.2), and can also be benchmarked when looking at the provision in place particularly for individuals who have had previous trauma in their lives. Each of these elements allow people the opportunity to develop mutual relationships and to have their emotional experiences responded to appropriately.

- Does the behaviour threaten to break, damage or stress load our working relationship?
- Do I feel hostile or ambivalent to the person I am working with?
- Is and earlier patter of rejection and relationship breakdown happening again?
- Does the person seem fearful, unsure of how to react to me or show strange behaviours?
- Do I feel emotionally unavailable or cut off from the person?

Figure 8.2: Relational risk questions (Skelly, 2014)

These elements fit with ideas of emotionally aware care as described in some detail by Shackleton (2016). This describes how stable and secure relationships can be provided for people in paid care environments, through the provision of a core staff team. This team needs to provide 'good-enough care', which is attuned, consistent, reliable and nurturing, while holding boundaries. Many of these aims can be explicitly linked to PBS aims of ensuring that staff have a clear plan about how to provide support at different stages of the time-intensity model, and that this occurs in a predictable and consistent way across the team. The PBS plan can outline some of these elements and allow thought to be given to the practicalities for providing a core team, such as considering the challenges of staff burn-out or being overwhelmed by the client's emotional needs. Other practical considerations include shift length, rotations and breaks. Emotional well-being of staff can also be enhanced by team formulation, understanding which boundaries to hold, as well as providing the staff team with time for reflection. This should include recognising any parallel processes about power and powerlessness, and responding to these if necessary. These will all help reduce staff burn-out.

Finally, central to PBS is the understanding of people's behavioural presentation. The assessment, functional analysis and formulation of behaviour should be central to the interventions. This is also the case for trauma-related understandings of behaviour as we look to understand behaviour as a symptom of distress and to connect within a relationship ensuring "…good enough care which is reliable, containing, empathetic and attuned" (Hughes, 2016).

Triggers and functions of behaviours through a trauma-informed lens

The focus on 'functions of behaviour' in PBS means that it is accepted that behaviours that are challenging serve a purpose to the person engaging in them – that purpose develops due to the person's experiences and continues as it serves a helpful function to the person. It is important that when assessing for behaviours that challenge, we incorporate assessments in relation to trauma, as outlined in earlier chapters. In trauma-informed terms, we would think of behaviours that challenge as the person's best way of coping – that the behaviour developed in response to the trauma, and made sense at the time of the trauma. In addition, it is well documented that there are neurological changes relating to trauma in childhood that can remain present in adulthood. These changes lead to people being hypervigilant to danger, more responsive to danger clues, less aware of safety cues and quicker to respond to perceived danger. The neurological aspects of trauma, including hyperarousal to danger and/or reduction in understanding of safety cues, are also key to understanding trauma within a PBS framework. To put this into terminology of PBS, people with intellectual disabilities who have also experienced complex trauma are more likely to notice danger, so have more slow triggers that can lead to escalation. They are also likely to escalate quickly to crisis, as they are more likely to use quick neurological processing (via the amygdala) than the slower hippocampus routes. If people have more of an avoidant attachment style, then they may show more withdrawn behaviours, which can be less challenging but may still benefit from a trauma-informed explanation.

In assessing the function of behaviours for individuals with trauma backgrounds, we need to look beyond the short-term functions of behaviour that may be in place (escape/avoidance; social attention; seeking tangible reinforcers; sensory seeking or automatic behaviours), and think about the longer-term elements of reinforcement that may be operating for people (Patterson, 2016). Patterson (2016) discusses these longer-term maintaining functions of behaviour. For instance, he argues we need to look at how behaviours that challenge allow the individual to assert control or power, in otherwise powerless situations (e.g. Harding and Fisher, 2009). We also need to recognise how behaviours that challenge can serve the function of keeping others at 'arm's length', thus reducing opportunity for relationship building and skill development. In extreme circumstances this can include the implementation of seclusion or isolated care for long periods of time, meaning that they do not have opportunities to engage in relationships in any way. When relationships have been painful at best and abusive at worst, it can make some sense why engagement is avoided. However, without this engagement we cannot help people to develop relational and emotional skills. In addition, this has further implications for the individual's self-esteem and sense of self, and trauma-related responses are reinforced as well as the narratives that an individual has about themselves and that others have about them.

In addition, as people are hypervigilant to threats, then good behavioural management is about helping staff to be calm and reflective in the way they approach and interact with people – even moving closer could be threatening (Fowler, 2020). Equally, many of the triggers are internal for people who have had trauma. They are about their emotional and relational experiences, and so may be more complicated to observe (whereas external triggers are more easily observed). Helping staff to reflect and respond to these involves self-reflection and acknowledgment of one's own feelings about supporting individuals – helping people to implement the emotional containment outlined within a PBS plan.

Furthermore, it can be complicated for staff to provide support to individuals who might seem unengaged or sabotaging of help, or whom might show big emotional reactions to seemingly small events (Hughes, 2016). This in turn can lead to staff becoming disengaged or unresponsive to emotional needs. This is similar to the notion of 'blocked care' used in dyadic behaviour psychotherapies, meaning that when you block the capacity for delight you also block the capacity for rejection (Hughes, 2016). When staff feel overwhelmed it is understandably hard to know what to offer. Equally, it can be distressing or scary to work with individuals with high levels of behaviours that challenge (Whitby, 2008). There is a risk then that staff approach individuals in a way that can be a trigger, as summarised in this quote:

'If someone approaches me for a conversation and they are full of worry, fear or anger, I find myself suddenly in the same state of emotion.'

– Attwood & Garnett, 2016

Through understanding these relational triggers and longer-term functions of behaviour, we can begin to explore proactive ways of intervening and allow people to have these functions met in healthier and developmentally appropriate ways. This will enable individuals to develop skills in these areas to gain appropriate power and control in their lives, as well as services avoiding responding in an inappropriate or re-traumatising way.

Including trauma-informed ideas within a PBS plan

So, PBS fits alongside TIC, and now I will directly link each element of a standard PBS layout. The format used is based upon the iPBS plans (Nethal *et al.,* 2015). The aim is to show how trauma-based interventions can be linked within this framework.

My best day

'My best day' is a section of the PBS plan, which includes the person's preferred daily routine and their enjoyable activities etc. Very often this is written with the person and always with people who know them well. There may be opportunity in here to talk about the elements of trauma and hyper arousal, and how these can be managed. If relationships are difficult, then thinking about this in this section can be helpful too.

Understanding my behaviour

It is important that we encompass the trauma-informed understandings of the person's presentation; how their lack of understanding of safety cues, their hypervigilance to danger and their best ways of coping, are now seen as behaviours that challenge. In addition, how working proactively we can help them reach a window of tolerance and optimal operational zone (Ogden, 2015). Through these ideas, we aim to help them engage in fewer behaviours that challenge and enable a move towards a better quality of life, which obviously needs to be individually tailored.

Understanding relational dynamics can also form a part of this formulation and includes helping staff teams to reflect on their own emotional responses to the support they are offering. This can in turn connect with their own histories (including trauma histories) and having time and space to do this needs to be a priority in ensuring services can provide that secure base. Using forums such as case workshops (Hill and Harding, 2019) and team formulation (e.g. Lake, 2008) can enable people to reflect on their experiences and to deepen their understanding of what support the individual with intellectual disability needs. This is rarely a one-off occurrence but needs to be revisited, through fortnightly or monthly staff reflection sessions and look at incidents and day-to-day interactions.

Primary prevention strategies

In the multi-element model of behavioural interventions, different proactive strategies are proposed in terms of ecological strategies, learning new skills and focused support (LaVinga and Willis, 2015). Each of these can be examined through a trauma lens; aiming to increase the quality of the person's relationship by skilling carers up in their interactions. In Crates *et al's.* (2013) work they have explicitly linked behavioural theory with trauma approaches, and to a range of interventions from within the trauma-informed model, summarised in Table 8.1.

Table 8.1:Mapping trauma strategies to the Multi-element model (MEM)			
Proactive strategies			Reactive strategies
Ecological strategies	Learning new skills	Focused support	
Physical Low arousal sensory strategies **Interpersonal** Attachment – theory – interpersonal relationships are critical Attunement and co-regulation Life-story therapy **Programmatic** Consistent, predictable and patterned repeated experiences	Play therapy Dyadic development psychotherapy Cognitive behavioural therapy Dialectical behaviour therapy Life-story therapy Eye movement desensitisation and reprocessing Mindfulness Psycho-education **Explicit teaching strategies for staff to follow: shaping, fading.**	**Managing antecedents** Attunement and co-regulation Low arousal sensory strategies **Differential schedules** Suppressing problems and engaging with services	**Non-functionally based** Attunement and co-regulation Low arousal sensory strategies **Functionally based** *Traditional methods – (not recommended in the MEM*)* ** – might be considered last resort*
Mediators Attunement and co-regulation Mindfulness Blocked care Parallel process Shared framework Shared language Consistency TIC Biopsychosocial approach to understanding Action affect awareness Non-linear understanding			

In the physical environment, helping individuals develop better skills to manage their needs, particularly in relation to interpersonal interactions, can draw on ideas from the circle of security literature; where staff hold the position of secure base, allowing people to explore and experiment but to be safe and welcomed on return (for ideas regarding application of circle of security see Schuengel *et al.,* 2016).

This can take many months, even years, for people who have been 'miscued' about safety in the past. Strategies in relation to building and maintaining relationships are also important to help carers to not be pulled into blocked care interactions and to ensure the capability for repair and reflection within relationships. Part of this relational skill building includes the idea of rewarding what you want to see and allowing space for mistakes to be reflected upon. There is scope to skill people up in relational skills and in their emotional regulation skills (using ideas from other models, such as Dialectical Behaviour Therapy (DBT). The trust in relationships and the ability to be soothed by the presence of another, are a part of this development.

Antecedents management can be thought about and relational elements discussed with the person where that is possible, including explanations and clear boundaries about staff shift patterns, leaving shift and post.

To aid with these interventions within the PBS plan, there may also be a statement about how this helps to develop the person build a secure relationship (Skelly, 2016) or how this aids them in operating in the optimal arousal zone. It is through the development of the secure base that we will enable people to be able to access other proactive strategies (such as some of the individual therapies).

In addition, it can be useful to think of the areas of behaviour presentation outlined in Figure 8.1, where, due to trauma, these developmental skills have not been developed yet or behaviours have developed to help the person cope, but which are no longer helpful. Using interventions that aid these skills within a developmental perspective can be helpful. Proactive skills that aid the development of these other areas may include understanding the shield of shame (Golding and Hughes, 2012), being able to reflect on behaviours (behavioural chains; Linehan, 1993) to build skills in prediction of events, intensive interaction to build turn-taking skills (Nind and Hewitt, 2001), or increase sense of control and conversational games to aid with development of self and exploration of safe differences between people.

It is useful to consider Golding's (2015) pyramid model of meeting the needs of traumatised children in stages by which they might need to progress, when applying this to staff teams supporting adults with trauma histories. This is adapted and presented in Table 8.2. The primary preventative strategies of the PBS plan could consider meeting the elements of the stages outlined in the table.

Table 8.2: based upon Golding's work for traumatised children but conceptualised for staff teams	
Stage one	Established relationships with the care/staff team – using clear boundaries and crisis plans
Stage two	Embed these relationships – using ideas around repair and ensuring all elements of emotional security for the individual, staff and multi-disciplinary team
Stage three	Help further develop emotional coping skills and more adaptive responses to feelings of distress, which may help reduce behaviours that challenge
Stage four	To continue providing this for the long-term. To enabling individuals to continue to use their emotional coping and relationship-forming skills to develop relationships within their staff team and communities.

Secondary Preventative strategies

Secondary preventative strategies need to include the trauma strategies that are helpful when people become over-aroused emotionally due to lack of soothing skills. These can include grounding techniques and sensory activities to help the person return to an optimal zone of functioning. As always with trauma and increased distress, there is a risk that the problem-solving part of the brain could be likened to being 'off-line' as people become more emotionally aroused (PODS, 2018), so thinking about presenting things visually or with a demonstration to reduce the verbal processing rather than asking people about this can be helpful within the PBS plan. It is unlikely people will be able to self-sooth, and yet we must not assume that the presence of another is inherently soothing (Hughes, 2016). Being aware of triggers relating to interactions and lack of safety are part of the trauma-informed understandings of the person and their likely escalation. Using ideas within a PACE approach (Playful, Accepting, Curious and Empathetic; Golding and Hughe, 2012) about being tentatively curious about increased distress, naming emotions and possible triggers, may help a person to understand their reactions (see chapter 10). This approach can also enhance staff's understanding of the triggers to the persons' distress.

It is also relevant that carers understand the triggers of behaviour and the function of behaviour (short- and long-term) to offer with the aim of de-escalating the person's emotional distress prior to them reaching crisis if and where feasible.

Reactive strategies

Using a PBS framework, it is possible to be clear about relational goals. When working with individuals who have reached crisis point it remains important to hold boundaries. It may however not be the time to explain these or contracts that are pre-agreed when the individual is on baseline. It is also important that any ruptures in relationship repair are thought about and modelled by staff. At these times of crisis, holding the emotional security is important, to help the person feel understood and safe to experience overwhelming feelings.

A crisis plan does need to be developed to ensure that people feel safe, for both the person who has experienced previous trauma and their carers currently offering care. Otherwise, the relational security elements are not fulfilled. Ultimately, we are moving people to a place of emotional security though their relationship, not their environment, but this will take time.

If we do not think about TIC, there is a risk of re-traumatising

There are also risks of not considering trauma in providing support packages – that in not providing some of the elements above we risk re-traumatising individuals. There are reasons why being in long-term care places individuals at risk of repeated trauma and lack of attachments. These include the following elements according to the BPS (2017):

- frequent changes in staff personnel, which prevents the development of meaningful relationships and interrupts or blocks opportunities for repair.

- high workload of staff: as well as volume of workload there is also often an emphasis on elements other than 'good quality care' and the type of relationship, and yet relationships need to be given priority and be captured and evaluated so that they can impact on good quality care.

- discontinuity of staff presence: and often that there will be more staff support during incidents of behaviours that challenge, which can be reinforcing or overwhelming and needs to be thought about in relation to how staff are deployed to work with people and how their time is prioritised.

- limited opportunities for individual support – which again impacts on the development of individuals one-to-one relationships, which are attuned to individual need and emotional responses.

- organisational cultures that value independence from staff rather than mutual interdependence – and that increased independence and autonomy for clients/people with an ID may become a focus too soon, within an attachment perspective, and where those clients still need interdependence and meaningful relationships in order to develop.

- lack of support for paid carers in negotiating relationship boundaries.

Relational security, emotionally aware care, core teams and explicit facilitation of reflection on the emotional elements of providing care to those who have experienced trauma, can minimise staff burn-out, which can reduce frequent changes in staff personal. As Whitby (2008) recognises staff will do what the organisation is seen to value, and often this is paperwork-based. However, if it is relationships or provision of the conditions of security that the organisation values then staff are more likely to prioritise this (in PBS positive monitoring can be adapted to look at this). In addition, this can aid with planning opportunities for staff to have individual support with people which can be limited in busy environments. Behaviours that challenge can be a way for people to access increased one-to-one time. However, that might be reduced if people's behaviour improves. Understanding this from a trauma and coping perspective can aid with this for the individual, their staff team and at a wider organisational level.

Cultures within ID services might value independence over interdependence; which means that people are not being provided with emotionally aware care or opportunities for shared mutual explorations and enjoyment. There can be a lack of support and guidance about how paid carers are meant to be negotiating relationships and their own emotional responses. Relationships are an important component within all PBS plans. However, when these are particularly tricky due to previous responses to trauma, a PBS plan can enhance and support the staff team to consider relational styles and approaches that will best help the presenting issues. Sharing the ideas of blocked care and blocked trust can aid in staff remembering that these relational difficulties are not personal to them, and reinforce the need to connect before correct (Hughes, 2016).

In addition, one of the most re-traumatising experiences for people that have had trauma in their lives can be the use of restraint, (e.g. Heyvaert et al., 2014). Despite pledges to reduce restriction, statistics have shown that the number of restrictive interventions used in inpatient units on people with intellectual disabilities increased from the years 2016 to 2018, with the largest increase being in physical restraints (BBC, 2019). It is highly possible that this is re-traumatising for people and so needs to be thought about incredibly carefully. There is therefore a need to be actively planning to reduce restraint usage for individuals and this needs, therefore, to incorporate proactive ways of supporting people and responding to their distress. So again, the goals of PBS are directly related to the goals of TIC and ensuring that the person is offered relationships that are caring, compassionate and empathetic, with the aim of reducing restrictive practices.

Sadly, in services there are often examples of relationships that are intended to be caring, but become traumatic for individuals with an ID. In some cases, this is due to explicitly unacceptable behaviour from carers (as seen in scandals such as Winterbourne View and Walton Hall in the UK). However, this is often, related to complex relationships with power and the repeated cycle of power not being placed with individuals with ID, or their families (see Oakes, 2012). Using PBS to reflect on these power imbalances and addressing them with staff teams and across organisations can also be critical.

The PBS approach, combined with trauma-informed approaches and operating with compassionate leadership, can be the vehicle by which TIC can be operationalised in the lives of people with behaviours that challenge. It places emphasis on what staff need to do to ensure that meaningful relationships and attunement to emotional need are placed centrally. If the PBS framework can take a trauma-informed approach, then the principles of TIC, safety, empowerment, choice, collaboration and trust can be central and explicit within PBS plans. They sit alongside the PBS components of choice, community presence, respect, relationships and goals of increasing quality of life and reducing emotional distress. Furthermore, if the function of behaviours is reflective of a person's trauma history, and this is incorporated into understanding the person and their behaviours that challenge, this allows interventions in relation to trauma recovery to be realised for individuals and at a wider organisational level.

References

Allan, D, (2009). Positive behavioural support as a service system for people with challenging behaviour. *Psychiatry*, **8**(10), 408-412.

Attwood T & Garnett M (2016) *Exploring Depression and Beating the Blues: A CBT self-help guide to understanding and coping with depression in Asperger's syndrome [ASD-Level 1].* Jessica Kingsley Publishers, London, UK.

BBC News (2019) *The failings in learning disability services in six charts* [online]Available at: https://www.bbc.co.uk/news/health-48355111 (accessed 17 September 2020)

BILD, NHS Health Education England, Skills for Care, Challenging Behaviour Foundation & PBS Academy (2017) *Key messages about positive behavioural support* [online]. Available at: http://pbsacademy.org.uk/wp-content/uploads/2017/05/PBS-key-messages-April-2017-1.pdf (accessed 10 October 2020).

BPS (2017) *Incorporating Attachment Theory into Practice: Clinical practice guideline for clinical psychologists working with people who have intellectual disabilities.* Leicester: BPS.

Coles, S and Ellis-Caird, H. 2019. Whose story is it anyway? A narrative approach to working with people affect by learning disabilities, their families and Networks. In: V Jones & M Hayton-Laurelut (Eds) *Working with People with Learning Disabilities: Systemic approaches*. London, UK: Red Globe Press.

Crates N, Spicer M, Burton & Pullen, 2013. *Trauma Informed Support for People with Disability* [online]. Available at: https://www.asid.asn.au/files/219_24_n_crates_m_spicer.pdf file:///C:/Users/cathy.harding/AppData/Local/Microsoft/Windows/INetCache/Content.Outlook/B450ZFBK/Crates%20Trauma%20Informed%20Support%20for%20People%20with%20Disability%20(003).pdf. (Accessed 10th December 2020).

Fisher C & Harding C (2009) Thoughts on the rebel role: Its application to challenging behaviour in learning disability services. *Reformulation* Summer 4–8.

Fowler S (2020) Understanding Behaviours of Concern through a Polyvagal Lens. BILD Virtual Positive Behavioural Support Conference, September 29, 30 and 1 October 2020.

Golding K (2015) *Meeting the therapeutic needs of traumatized children* [online]. Available at: https://kimsgolding.co.uk/resources/models/meeting-the-therapeutic-needs-of-traumatized-children/ (accessed 10 December 2020).

Golding K & Hughes D (2012) *Creating Loving Attachments: Parenting with PACE: To nurture confidence and security in the trouble child*. London: Jessica Kingsley.

Heyvaert M, Saenen L, Maes B & Onghena P (2014) Systematic review of restraint interventions for challenging behaviour among persons with intellectual disabilities: Focus on effectiveness in single case experiments. *Journal of Applied Research in Intellectual Disabilities* **27**(6) 493-510.

Hill C & Harding C (2019) Working systemically with multi-disciplinary teams. In: V Jones & M Hayton-Laurelut (Eds) *Working with People with Learning Disabilities: Systemic approaches*. London, UK: Red Globe Press.

Hughes, D. (2016) How early years trauma affects the brain of a child who mistrusts good care [online]. Available at: https://www.youtube.com/watch?v=xuRagD9ES9w {accessed 7 December 2020).

Jackson AL & Waters SE (2015) *Taking Time – Framework: A trauma-informed framework for supporting people with intellectual disability*. Melbourne, Australia: Berry Street.

Kezeler C & Stravropoulos P (2012) *The Last frontier: Practice Guidelines for Trauma Informed Care and Service Delivery. Adults surviving sexual abuse* [online]. Available at: https://www.childabuseroyalcommission.gov.au/sites/default/files/IND.0521.001.0001.pdfwww.asca.org.au.

Lake N (2008). Developing skills in consultation 2: A team Formulation approach. *Clinical psychology Forum* **186**, 18-24.

LaVinga GW & Willis T (2015) A Positive Behavioural Support Model for Breaking the Barriers to Social and Community Inclusion. *Tizard Learning Disability Review* **10** (2) 16-23.

Linehan M (1993) Cognitive-Behavioural Treatment of Borderline Personality Disorder (diagnosis and Treatment of mental disorders). New York: Guilford Press.

Nethel G, Smith M, Lowe K & Jones E (2015) *Individual Positive Behavioural Support Plan (IPBS) format*. Specialist Behavioural Team, Learning Disabilities and Mental health Delivery unit, Swansea Bay Health Board. Nind M & Hewitt D (2001) A practical guide to intensive interaction. Kidderminster: BILD.

NICE (2015). *Challenging behaviour and learning disabilities: prevention and interventions for people with learning disabilities whose behaviour challenges*. https://www.nice.org.uk/guidance/ng11 (retrieved 22nd March 2021)

Oakes P (2012) Crash: What went wrong at Winterbourne View? *Journal of Intellectual Disabilities* **16** (3) 155-162.

O'Brien J (1992) Developing high quality services for people with developmental disabilities. In: VJ Bradley & HA Bersane (Eds) *Quality Assurance for Individuals with Developmental Disabilities*. Baltimore: Paul Brookes.Ogden P. (2015) Sensorimotor Psychotherapy: Interventions for Trauma and Attachment. London, UK: WW Norton and Co.

Patterson (2016) *Attachment Trauma and relationships*. One day training. BILD

PODS (2018). Three parts of the Brain: Impairments during the 'suicidal mode'. Dealing with distress, working with self harm and suicide. Bristol.

RCP, BPS, RCSLT (2007) *Challenging Behaviour: A Unified Approach*. Leicester: BPS.

Schuengel C, Clegg J, Clasien de Schipper J & Kef S (2016) Adult attachment and care staff functioning. In: HK Fletcher, A Flood & DJ Hare (Eds) *Attachment and Intellectual and Developmental Disability. A Clinicians Guide to Practice and Research*. Chichester: Wiley.

Shalketon A (2016) Have a Heart: Helping Services to Provide Emotionally Aware Support. In: HK Fletcher, A Flood & DJ Hare (Eds) *Attachment and Intellectual and Developmental Disability. A Clinicians Guide to Practice and Research*. Chichester: Wiley.

Skelly A (2014). *Attachment Trauma and relationships*. One day training. BILD.

Skelly A (2016) Maintaining the bond: working with people who are described as Showing Challenging Behaviour Using a Framework Based on Attachment Theory. In: HK Fletcher, A Flood & DJ Hare (Eds) *Attachment and Intellectual and Developmental Disability. A Clinicians Guide to Practice and Research*. Chichester: Wiley.

Spring C (2019) *Recovery is possible*. Podcast # 2 [online]. https://www.carolynspring.com/podcasts/ (accessed 1 December 2020).

Spring C (2019) Can we heal? Podcast #7 [online]. Available at: https://www.carolynspring.com/podcasts/ (accessed 1 December 2020). Whitby (2008) Why is good quality residential care so very very difficult to achieve? *Journal of dementia care* March/April 2008 30-33.

Chapter 9:
The use of Intensive Interaction in trauma-informed care for people with severe and profound intellectual disabilities

Judith Samuel and Sophie Doswell

Introduction

For people with severe or profound intellectual disabilities (ID), the recognition and response to the experience of trauma presents additional challenges. Services may themselves be experienced as traumatic or re-traumatising. Intensive Interaction is not a specific trauma approach. However, it is useful both proactively and as an intervention within the context of trauma-informed care (TIC).

Of the population of people with ID (American Psychiatric Association, 2013), 3-4 per cent are described as having severe ID. This group has basic levels of communication and needs daily supervision and support. Whereas 1-2 per cent of the population are described as having profound ID. This group has extremely limited communication ability and depends on others for all aspects of day-to-day life. Individuals with severe and profound ID present with uneven profiles of cognitive deficits in perception, memory and information-processing, exacerbated by extremely slow developmental progress. They are more likely to have sensory impairments and sensory processing difficulties, physical disabilities and serious medical conditions. Having multiple complex needs particularly applies to people with the most significant ID (Doukas *et al.*, 2017).

Are people with severe and profound ID more at risk of trauma than those with milder ID?

Exposure to adverse life events and environmental stressors is high for people with ID, and may result in psychological and physical health problems (Wigham and Emerson, 2015; Marcal and Trifoso, 2017). There is some evidence that such exposure is disproportionately experienced by individuals with severe and profound ID. Hershkowitz *et al.* (2007) found in a review of records that severity of ID was associated with both increased incidence of abuse and degree of harm compared with typically developing children. Reasons for this may include the view by abusers that such victims would be unable to report what had happened and be considered less credible (Manders and Stoneman, 2009).

People with severe or profound ID are unlikely to have sufficient control over their environment to avoid triggers relating to past trauma (Wigham and Emerson, 2015). Individuals may not be able to seek explicit support to regulate their distress and any withdrawal as a response to trauma may be overlooked. They may have learned repeated patterns of behaviour as ways to self-soothe or to manage emotional distress in the context of an unsafe and unpredictable external world. Such coping behaviours may become labelled as challenging and/or signs of mental health difficulties (Doukas *et al.*, 2017) and even result in restrictive responses (medication, restraint, seclusion or institutionalisation), which are also experienced as traumatic (Singh *et al.*, 2016).

Services as a source of trauma for people with severe and profound ID

From the late 1960s onward, UK service philosophy based on normalisation/social role valorisation (Wolfensberger,1972; 1983) focused on breaking the vicious circle of prejudiced belief, low expectations, opportunity deprivation, negative experience and decreased performance (O'Brien and Tyne, 1981). Under the Education [Handicapped Children] Act (1970), people with severe and profound

ID previously considered 'uneducable' (Education Act, 1944) could attend school. It was intended that all people with ID would lead an 'ordinary life' (Kings Fund, 1982). Nonetheless, compared with the more able, people with severe and profound ID were still missing out on having their needs met (Raynes, 1980). Coffman and Harris (1980) described the transition shock and adjustment difficulties associated with de-institutionalisation. For someone with severe or profound ID, moving out of an institution meant losing familiar staff, environments and routines. Oswin (1991) describes how the trauma of bereavement and loss was being neglected. People with the most significant ID were thought not to notice or to understand these changes, yet, at the same time, carers expressed concerns about individuals' unmanageable distress. Even within the newly created specialist community services, the needs of those with more significant impairments were found to be marginalised: in day services (e.g. Rose *et al.,* 1993) and at home (e.g. Perry and Felce, 1994), institutionalisation still occurred, often a long way from home.

'Age appropriateness', a key idea of normalisation/social role valorisation, refers to 'social expectations, opportunities and experiences' (O'Brien and Tyne, 1981) typical for a chronological age and culture. It was predicted that if adults with ID were no longer treated as children they would gain adult competencies, a more accepted social image (Porter, Grove and Park, 1996) and self-esteem (Calhoun and Calhoun, 1993). However, such research did not explore these outcomes for people with severe or profound ID. Instead, Bartlett and Bunning (1997) described the damaging cycle of 'over estimation', the impact of unrealistic expectations resulting in an individual withdrawing emotionally and communicating even less, and the system around them trying even harder but in inappropriate ways to meet needs. Doing nothing through fear of criticism for not being age-appropriate also occurred. People with profound ID were termed 'the ignored minority', even within a specialist ID service (Samuel and Pritchard, 2001).

Challenges from services for people with more significant ID continue. For example, Emerson and Baines (2010) reported the mortality rate for individuals with 'moderate to severe' ID was three times higher than for the general population due to a range of avoidable health difficulties. Despite governmental demand for improvements following scandals (Department of Health, 2012) institutional abuse has continued in services for people with ID (e.g. Murphy, 2020; Muckamore Abbey Hospital Review Team, 2020) where, even though not explicitly stated, some of the victims living in these institutions are likely to have a severe or profound ID.

The COVID-19 pandemic has brought new triggers. The distress for people with severe and profound ID caused by sudden changes of routine and relationships, and being supported by family and other carers who themselves are experiencing trauma is likely to be great. The negative impact on communication and emotional well-being of 'social distancing', the use of masks without mouths showing and the wearing of other personal protective equipment should not be underestimated.

Identifying trauma within people with severe and profound ID

Adapted self-report post-traumatic stress disorder (PTSD) measures are inappropriate for use with individuals with severe and profound ID. Informant versions of measures (Wigham *et al.,* 2011) and observation schedules, either idiosyncratically designed (Bakken *et al.,* 2014) or published (Frankish, 2019), may be used. A thorough review of historical records is required, although these may not always be freely available or contain sufficient detail. Informants with knowledge of an individual's history are helpful, but may not always exist as staff turnover can be high and family contact minimal or non-existent, leaving some individuals with severe and profound ID without anyone holding their history and any stories of harmful experiences.

Trauma may be overlooked as a predictor of behaviours that challenge (Wigham and Emerson, 2015). Bakken *et al.* (2014) describe how an inpatient with severe ID and a diagnosis of psychosis showed signs of extreme arousal whenever a nap was suggested. It was discovered that he had been the victim of belt restraint and seclusion. Developing an understanding of this individual's behaviour in the context of previous traumatic experiences allowed for his diagnosis of psychosis to be reconsidered and removed and a trauma-informed care plan to be introduced.

Signs of trauma in individuals with severe or profound ID may include:
> *'strange reactions to everyday situations, using actions or words they did not use before, withdrawal from others or clinging to someone, and an increase in challenging behaviour. For example, someone who was restrained on the floor regularly now lies down on the floor when an incident escalates.'*
> – Challenging Behaviour Foundation [CBF], n.d.

The network around an individual with severe or profound ID (including families, staff and professionals) therefore, has a responsibility for identifying both potentially traumatic experiences and changes in behaviour that suggest a traumatic reaction to those experiences. It is only once trauma is suspected or identified that appropriate responses can be planned and implemented.

Constructive responses to trauma for people with severe and profound ID

Skelly's (2017) Conditions for Security model describes the importance of emotional availability and predictability, warmth, mutual enjoyment and shared exploration in developing attachment. Interactions with, and services for, individuals with severe and profound ID should meet these conditions for security, to build positive attachments within relationships that can be protective for individuals if there are difficult experiences in the future. Caregiver responses need to be attuned to the attachment needs of the individual, whether or not behaviours of concern are present.

TIC for individuals with ID includes (Marcal and Trifoso, 2017):

- training on recognising trauma and its impact
- promotion of carer self-care
- restorative, rather than re-traumatising, responses.

Singh *et al.* (2016) acknowledge that well-trained staff who have been taught mindfulness as self-care, are much less likely to resort to physical intervention. Marcal and Trifoso (2017) present a trauma-informed support plan for a man with profound ID, autism and PTSD. This includes relationship building, reducing restrictive interventions, enabling safety, empowerment and minimising unexpected change. The plan is also explicit about the therapeutic place of physical touch.

Intensive Interaction in TIC

Why Intensive Interaction is relevant in TIC

Intensive Interaction can be used to help individuals with severe or profound ID to reduce the likelihood of trauma and re-trauma through the development of relationships. The emotional benefits of Intensive Interaction (Hewett, 2018) match the interactional features in Skelly's Conditions for Security model. Intensive Interaction aims to help participants feel seen and understood, it is empowering and (re)builds connection, safety and pleasurable experiences. In addition, Intensive Interaction can be utilised as part of a restorative therapeutic approach when an individual has experienced trauma.

What is Intensive Interaction?

Intensive Interaction is an approach that enhances the responsiveness of caregivers to support people with ID and/or autism who are functioning at the early levels of human interaction. It aims to develop fundamental interactional abilities: how to communicate and to enjoy being with others (Nind and Hewett, 2005; Intensive Interaction Institute website).

The basis for Intensive Interaction is the view that early learning occurs within a dynamic social context (Schaffer 1977; Stern, 1977). Both infant and caregiver initiate interaction and imitate each other with mutual enjoyment. The infant develops a sense of self and agency and the dyad learns that they can turn take, influence each other and share meaning. Familiarity, emotional security and attachment grow (Bowlby, 1971).

Intensive Interaction began in the 1980s within an educational establishment of a long-stay hospital near London (Nind and Hewett, 2005). The principles that Intensive Interaction draws on from early caregiver-infant interaction are outlined by Nind and Hewett (2001):

- 'being available
- being observant and tuned in
- being responsive
- relaxing and enjoying the interaction
- being warm and playful
- celebrating responses and new behaviours
- allowing pauses
- letting the…person…lead
- creating and repeating familiar enjoyable interactions
- extending your responses to become turn-taking and other new developments.'

In practice, Intensive Interaction differs in detail for each participant as it is based upon their individual interests and presentation. It may involve the practitioner using eye contact, mirroring breathing patterns, vocalisations or facial expressions, repeating physical movements such as tapping or rocking, or sharing interest in sensory or play items.

The evidence base for Intensive Interaction

Intensive Interaction has been described as having 'an emerging though limited evidence base' (Baker, 2015), although the quality of reporting has been criticised (Hutchinson and Bodicoat, 2015). See Firth (2019) for a comprehensive summary of the latest evidence. Of relevance to TIC, gains have been reported in social engagement and rapport (Nind, 1996; Watson and Fisher, 1997; Kellett, 2000; 2003; 2004; Cameron and Bell, 2001; Anderson, 2006; Barber, 2008; Samuel *et al.,* 2008; Zeedyk *et al.,* 2009; Zeedyk, Caldwell and Davies, 2009; Argyropoulou and Papoudi, 2012; Clegg *et al.,* 2018).

Nevertheless, research has yet to explore the direct impact of Intensive Interaction on the experience of trauma. Intensive Interaction has been noted as a useful approach to augment other interventions (British Psychological Society [BPS], 2016) and as a way of applying attachment in clinical practice for people with multiple and/or profound ID (BPS, 2017). Its use within all phases of a Positive Behaviour Support (PBS) plan (CBF, n.d.) is beginning to be described (McKim and Samuel, 2021).The use of Intensive Interaction is recommended in a range of UK service guidance including: Welsh Assembly Government (2006); Qualifications and Curriculum Authority (2009); Council for Curriculum, Examinations & Assessment (2011); Department of Health (2009; 2010); and Royal College of Speech and Language Therapists (2013).

Training in Intensive Interaction

Given its intuitive nature, Intensive Interaction does not require a formal practitioner qualification. Nevertheless, training opportunities are available supported by written guidance (e.g. Nind and Hewett, 2001; Hewett, 2018) and videos (e.g. Hewett, 2012). Research has demonstrated that even brief training can have a positive impact (Zeedyk *et al.,* 2009). To support ongoing learning, there is a passionate international community of practice (Barber and Firth, 2019; Intensive Interaction users Facebook group; Intensive Interaction Institute).

Implementing Intensive Interaction

Intensive Interaction is used by families, other carers and various professionals across education, health and social care settings. Anyone can start using Intensive Interaction. However, within a care setting, it is advised that its introduction incorporates the formal process of assessment, monitoring and reflection (Hewett and Nind, 1998; Nind and Hewett, 2001). The Mental Capacity Act (2005) states 'best interests' considerations must be addressed, and attention given to an individual's relationship history and complex needs. Use of social physical touch requires an organisational risk-management strategy (Hewett, 2007). Written and video records enable monitoring and support reflective practice. Scheduling sessions ensures priority is given and beginnings and endings planned. Nonetheless, opportunistic 'interactivity' (Nind and Hewett, 2005) is encouraged as part of everyday support and as a long-term strategy. A team approach is an essential protective factor against the loss of one significant attachment figure.

Relationship-building may occur through the informal, everyday use of Intensive Interaction by families and other carers. However, people with severe or profound ID who have a history of (institutional) abuse or loss may show behaviours of concern to such a degree (for example, screaming, throwing things, biting, spitting, smearing or sexualised behaviour) that it is hard for carers to build rapport by using this approach. Barriers to implementing Intensive Interaction include carers being hurt, worries about being seen as mocking individuals, perceiving that one is not doing things properly, managing endings, and struggling to integrate the approach with intimate and personal care. In this context, it is recommended that Intensive Interaction is introduced as a formal intervention delivered initially by an external experienced practitioner. Regular sessions develop a sense of safety in traumatised individuals and model the approach, providing a bridge to staff developing confidence in its more informal, everyday use.

Whether introduction of Intensive Interaction is informal or formal, sustainability must be addressed. Although rapport built via Intensive Interaction is, by definition, rewarding, and within a family context at least may become self-sustaining, maintenance, especially in the context of TIC, requires organisational commitment. Training for new carers, embedding in care plans, supporting reflective practice and evaluation of progress are all required (Barber and Firth, 2019). Regional practitioner peer supervision and support groups have developed (Nind and Hewett, 2001; Intensive Interaction Institute) and some organisations employ an Intensive Interaction co-ordinator/champion whose role is to lead on training, assessment, intervention, supporting reflective practice, monitoring and evaluation (Barber and Firth, 2019).

In any care setting, signs of physical pain, illness, neglect or abuse are expected to be addressed urgently. This meets Skelly's (2017) physical safety Conditions for Security. To meet the other conditions for security, it is recommended that Intensive Interaction should be considered an urgent proactive strategy when indicated by an individual's limited communication abilities and social environment (Doswell and Samuel, 2019).

Intensive Interaction in TIC: a case illustration

This case illustration is formed from a collation of work with individuals with severe and profound ID who have experienced trauma. Sereh (not her real name), a 66-year-old British woman of mixed heritage, was referred to the Community Learning Disabilities Team (CLDT) as she was pinching staff and visitors, and screaming. Her case was allocated to a clinical psychologist. Clinical psychologists in CLDTs will usually engage in a process of assessment, formulation (a testable idea or set of ideas about what is causing difficulties), intervention, and evaluation.

Assessment

The psychologist reviewed the records, interviewed staff and did some direct observation of day-to-day life. Sereh shared a residential home with five others where she had lived for over 10 years. At the age of 11, Sereh had been hospitalised because her family could no longer manage. Initially, her parents visited regularly but as Sereh showed distress when they left, they were advised to stop coming and forget her. She received limited schooling or opportunity to develop skills. She had acquired a visual impairment and, although records were unclear exactly how, this was thought to be a result of physical abuse by staff. Sereh appeared to have a profound ID, vocalised sounds and was physically able. She would curl up hugging herself for hours. Staff were reluctant to engage with Sereh to avoid the pinching and did not give her objects through fear she would throw them.

Three Intensive Interaction sessions occurred in the lounge in Sereh's favourite place, using vocalisations, physical mirroring and sensory objects. The aims were to identify Sereh's preferences and to build rapport. Sereh immediately became curious about the psychologist and made choices about the objects, throwing away what she did not prefer. She chose anything with which she could make a noise. She also delighted in action rhymes, such as 'Row, row, row your boat'.

Formulation

Sereh experienced grief from the sudden loss of her parents at a young age. She was one of many children in the institution, where, given low staff ratios, she would rarely have received one-to-one social engagement. She also suffered harm resulting in her visual impairment. These experiences would have made Sereh feel extremely unsafe. Her screaming and pinching seemed to be responses to trauma and the threat of re-trauma. She had learned that these behaviours kept potential perpetrators at bay and reduced the risk of her becoming close to people who may leave her, like her parents did. However, the present staff team had not considered that her current behaviour was trauma-related and simply tried to prevent it by keeping out of range and removing objects.

Intervention

The staff team were given brief training in TIC and Intensive Interaction, including Sereh's assessment and formulation. This was delivered in two separate two-hour sessions to capture the whole team. The focus was on helping staff to build rapport and trust through calm, consistent responses. To enhance Sereh's sense of safety and to model interaction for the staff, the psychologist offered 10 Intensive Interaction sessions. The psychologist also facilitated monthly reflective practice meetings to help the manager and staff team identify what was going well, and to consider the reasons for any challenges and to find solutions to them.

Outcomes

Over the Intensive Interaction sessions, rapport with the psychologist developed. Sereh became more engaged, willing to try new things and interested in what was happening around her. Following the training, staff began to notice signs that Sereh wanted interaction or did not and responded accordingly, so she did not have to use pinching to keep people away. They began to show delight in Sereh's enjoyment and felt less wary. Improved rapport meant staff offered Sereh sensory objects and the opportunity to be in the kitchen with them. Staff reported Sereh's screaming had reduced. Intensive Interaction was added to Sereh's support plan and sections updated in reflective practice meetings.

Sustainability

An Intensive Interaction champion was identified within the staff team. She received additional training and was allocated time to lead reflective practice, updating of the care plan and the induction of new staff using joint sessions and video feedback. She joined the local regional support group to help maintain her knowledge, skill and enthusiasm. After six months, the case was closed to the psychologist as Sereh was happier and more settled, and the service was well supported.

Conclusion

Families and services need to be aware that individuals with severe and profound ID are at least as likely to experience trauma as anyone else. Both historical information and current changes in behaviour are indicators of this. Services are embedding TIC that includes training, carer support and restorative responses. Intensive Interaction should be considered for use with people with severe and profound ID as a proactive strategy within PBS. Intensive Interaction aims to reduce the likelihood of further trauma as well as act as a restorative intervention. To implement Intensive Interaction, services require enough appropriately trained and supervised staff to offer person-centred support, to enable the development and maintenance of meaningful interactions and to build secure attachments. Services must create a positive social touch risk management strategy and enable ongoing reflective practice, monitoring and review, ideally using video feedback. Further research and service evaluation are required to explore Intensive Interaction's place in TIC, to ensure its appropriate and sustained use for individuals with severe and profound ID who would benefit from it.

Acknowledgements

Thank you to Mark Bryant and Jules McKim for help with literature searches.

References

American Psychiatric Association (APA) (2013) *Diagnostic and Statistical Manual of Mental Disorders* (5th edition). Arlington, Virginia: American Psychiatric Association.

Anderson C (2006) Early communication strategies: Using video analysis to support teachers working with preverbal pupils. *British Journal of Special Education* **33** (3) 114–120.

Argyropoulou Z & Papoudi D (2012) The training of a child with autism in a Greek preschool inclusive class through intensive interaction: A case study. *European Journal of Special Needs Education* **27** (1) 99–114.

Baker P (2015) Commentary on 'An audit of an Intensive Interaction service': *Tizard Learning Disability Review* **20** (3) 117–120.

Bakken TL, Kildahl AN, Gjersoe V, Matre E, Kristiansen T, Ro A, Tveter AL & Hoidal SH (2014) Identification of PTSD in adults with intellectual disabilities in five patients in a specialised psychiatric inpatient unit. *Advances in Mental Health and Intellectual Disabilities* **8** (2) 91–102.

Barber M (2008) Using intensive interaction to add to the palette of interactive possibilities in teacher-pupil communication. *European Journal of Special Needs Education* **23** (4) 393–402.

Barber M & Firth G (Eds) (2019) *Delivering Intensive Interaction Across Settings*. Melbourne: Independently published.

Bartlett C & Bunning K (1997) The importance of communication partnerships: A study to investigate the communicative exchanges between staff and adults with learning disabilities. *British Journal of Learning Disability* **25** 148-152.

Bowlby J (1969) *Attachment. Attachment and loss: Vol. 1. Loss*. New York: Basic Books.

British Psychological Society (2016) *Psychological therapies and people who have intellectual disabilities*. Leicester: British Psychological Society

British Psychological Society (2017) *Incorporating attachment theory into practice: clinical practice guideline for clinical psychologists working with people who have Intellectual Disabilities*. Leicester: British Psychological Society.

Calhoun ML & Calhoun LG (1993) Age-appropriate activities; Effects on the social perception of adults with mental retardation. *Education and Training in Mental Retardation* June 1993 143–148.

Cameron L & Bell D (2001) Enhanced interaction training: A method of multidisciplinary staff training in intensive interaction to reduce challenging behaviour in adults who have learning disabilities and who also have a severe communication disorder. *Working with People who have a Learning Disability* **18** (3) 8–15.

Challenging Behaviour Foundation (n.d.) *Positive Behaviour Support Planning: Part 3* [online]. Available at: https://www.challengingbehaviour.org.uk/learning-disability-files/03---Positive-Behaviour-Support-Planning-Part-3-web-2014.pdf (accessed August 2020).

Challenging Behaviour Foundation (n.d.) *Trauma FAQ* [online]. Available at: https://www.challengingbehaviour.org.uk/health-challenging-behaviour//trauma-support-faq.html (accessed August 2020).

Clegg J, Black R, Smith A & Brumfitt S (2018) Examining the impact of a city-wide intensive interaction staff training program for adults with profound and multiple learning disability: A mixed methods evaluation. *Disability and Rehabilitation* **42** (2) 201–210.

Coffman TL & Harris MC (1980) Transition shock and adjustments of mentally retarded persons. *Mental Handicap* **18** (1) 3–7.

Council for the Curriculum, Examinations and Assessment (2011) *Quest for learning: guidance and assessment materials – profound and multiple learning difficulties*. Belfast: Northern Ireland Council for Curriculum, Examinations and Assessment.

Department of Health (2009) *Valuing People Now*. London: Department of Health.

Department of Health (2010) *Raising our sights: Services for adults with profound intellectual and multiple disabilities*. London: Department of Health.

Department of Health (2012) *Transforming Care: A National Response to Winterbourne View Hospital*. London: Department of Health.

Doswell S & Samuel J (2019) *Intensive Interaction: A useful psychological approach within the frameworks of Positive Behaviour Support and Trauma Informed Care*. Paper presented at the BPS DCP FPID Annual Conference: London.

Doukas T, Fergusson A, Fullerton M & Grace J (2017) *Supporting People with Profound and Multiple Learning Disabilities: Core & essential service standards*. Northampton: PMLD Link.

Education Act (1944) (7 and 8 Geo 6 c. 31) London: United Kingdom Parliament.

Education [Handicapped Children] Act (1970) (c. 52) London: United Kingdom Parliament.

Emerson E & Baines S (2010) *Health Inequalities and People with Learning Disabilities in the UK*. Durham: Improving Health & Lives: Learning Disabilities Observatory.

Ephraim GW (1986) *A brief introduction to augmented mothering*. Playtrac Pamphlet, Radlett Herts: Harperbury Hospital.

Firth G (2019) *Intensive Interaction: The published research summaries document*. Leeds: Leeds and Yorks Partnership NHS Trust.

Frankish P (2019) *Frankish Assessment for the Impact of Trauma in Intellectual Disability*. Brighton: Pavilion Publishing.

Fulller PR (1949) Operant conditioning of a vegetative human organism. *American Journal of Psychology* **42** 587-590.

Gore NJ, McGill P, Toogood, S, Allen D, Hughes JC, Baker PA, Hastings RP, Noone SJ, Denne LD (2013) Definition and scope for positive behavioural support. *International Journal of Positive Behavioural Support* **3** (2) 14-23.

Hershkowitz I, Lamb ME & Horotiwitz D (2007) Victimisation of children with disabilities. *American Journal of Orthopsychiatry* **77** (4) 629-635.

Hewett D (2007) Do touch: Physical contact and people who have severe, profound and multiple learning difficulties. *Support for Learning* **22** (3) 116-123.

Hewett D (2012) *Intensive Interaction : So..what is Intensive Interaction* [online]. Available at: https://www.youtube.com/watch?v=gJruQPRx3Jk (accessed March 2021).

Hewett D (Ed) (2018) *The Intensive Interaction Handbook* (2nd edition). London: SAGE.

Hewett D & Nind M (Eds) (1998) *Interaction in Action: Reflection on the use of Intensive Interaction*. London: David Fulton.

Hutchinson N & Bodicoat A (2015) The effectiveness of Intensive Interaction: A systematic literature review. *Journal of Applied Research in Intellectual Disabilities* **28** 437-454.

Intensive Interaction Institute (n.d) [online]. Available at: https://www.intensiveinteraction.org (accessed September 2020).

Intensive Interaction Users Facebook Group (n.d) [online]. Available at: https://en-gb.facebook.com/groups/13657123715/ (accessed September 2020).

Kellett M (2000) Sam's story: Evaluating Intensive Interaction in terms of its effect on the social and communicative ability of a young child with severe learning difficulties. *Support for Learning* **15** (4) 165-171.

Kellett M (2003) Jacob's journey: Developing sociability and communication in a young boy with severe and complex learning difficulties using the Intensive Interaction teaching approach. *Journal of Research in Special Educational Needs* **3** (1) 18-34.

Kellett M (2004) Intensive Interaction in the inclusive classroom: Using interactive pedagogy to connect with students who are hardest to reach. *International Journal of Research & Method in Education* **27** (2) 175–88.

King's Fund Centre for Health Services Development (1982) *An Ordinary Life: Comprehensive locally-based residential services for mentally-handicapped people*. London: King's Fund.

Manders JE & Stoneman Z (2009) Children with disabilities in the child protective services system: An analog study of investigation and case management. *Child Abuse and Neglect* **33** 229-237.

Mansell J (2010) *Raising our Sights: Services for adults with profound intellectual and multiple disabilities*. London: Department of Health.

Marcal S & Trifoso S (2017) *A Trauma-Informed Toolkit for Providers in the Field of Intellectual & Developmental Disabilities* [online]. Available at: https://www.acesconnection.com/fileSendAction/fcType/0/fcOid/468137553002812476/filePointer/468137553002812517/fodoid/468137553002812512/IDD%20TOOLKIT%20%20CFDS%20HEARTS%20NETWORK%205-28%20FinalR2.pdf (accessed March 2021).

McGee JJ, Menolascino FJ, Hobbs DC & Menousek PE (1987) *Gentle Teaching: A non-aversive approach to helping persons with mental retardation*. New York: Human Science Press.

McKim J & Samuel J (2021) The use of Intensive Interaction within a Positive Behavioural Support Framework. *British Journal of Learning Disabilities*. **00**, 1-9

Mental Capacity Act (2005) (c.9) London: HMSO.

The Muckamore Abbey Review Team (2020) *A Review of leadership and governance at Muckamore Abbey Hospital* [online]. Available at: https://www.health-ni.gov.uk/sites/default/files/publications/health/doh-mah-review.pdf (Accessed August 2020).

Murphy, G (2020) *CQC inspections and regulation of Whorlton Hall 2015-2019: an independent review* [online]. CQC. https://www.cqc.org.uk/sites/default/files/20020218_glynis-murphy-review.pdf (accessed August 2020).

Nind M (1996) Efficacy of Intensive Interaction: Developing sociability and communication in people with severe and complex learning difficulties using an approach based on caregiver-infant interaction. *European Journal of Special Needs Education* **11** (1) 48-66.

Nind M & Hewett D (2001) *A Practical Guide to Intensive Interaction*. Kidderminster: BILD.

Nind M & Hewett D (2005) Access to Communication: Developing the basics of communication in people with severe learning difficulties through Intensive Interaction (2nd edition). London: David Fulton.

O'Brien J & Tyne A (1981) *The Principle of Normalisation: A foundation for effective services*. London: The Campaign for Mentally Handicapped People.

Oswin M (1991) *Am I Allowed to Cry? A study of bereavement amongst people who have learning difficulties*. London: Souvenir Press.

Perry J & Felce D (1994) Outcomes of ordinary housing services in Wales: Objective indicators. *Mental Handicap Research* **7** 286–311.

Porter J, Grove N & Park K (1996) Ages and stages. What is appropriate behaviour? In J Coupe O'Kane & J Goldbart (Eds) *Whose Choice? Contentious issues for those working with people with learning difficulties* (pp 58-69). London: David Fulton.

Qualifications and Curriculum Authority (2009) *Planning, teaching and assessing the curriculum for pupils with learning difficulties: general guidance*. London: QCA.

Raynes NV (1980) The less you've got the less you get: Functional groupings a cause for concern. *Mental Retardation* **28** 217–220.

Rose J, Davis C & Gotch L (1993) A comparison of the services provided to people with profound and multiple disabilities in two different day centres. *British Journal of Developmental Disabilities* **39** 83–94.

Royal College of Speech and Language Therapists (2013) *Five good communication standards*. London: RCSLT.

Samuel J, Nind M, Volans A & Scriven I (2008) An evaluation of Intensive Interaction in community living settings for adults with profound intellectual disabilities. *Journal of Intellectual Disabilities* **12** (2) 111-126.

Samuel J & Pritchard M (2001) The Ignored Minority: Meeting the needs of people with profound learning disability. *Tizard Learning Disability Review* **6** (2) 34–44.

Schaffer R (1977) *Mothering*. London: Fontana/Open Books.

Sharma V & Firth G (2012) Effective engagement through intensive interaction. *Learning Disability Practice* **15** (9) 20–23.

Singh NN, Lancioni GE, Karazsia BT, Chan J & Winton ASW (2016) Effectiveness of Caregiver Training in Mindfulness-Based Positive Behaviour Support (MBPBS) vs. Training-as-Usual (TAU): A Randomized Controlled Trial. *Frontiers in Psychology* **7** 1–13.

Skelly A (2017) Maintaining bonds: Positive behaviour support and attachment theory. *Clinical Psychology Forum* **290** 36–41.

Stern D (1977) *The First Relationship: Infant and mother*. London: Fontana/Open Books.

Watson J & Fisher A (1997) Evaluating the effectiveness of Intensive Interactive teaching with pupils with profound and complex learning difficulties. *British Journal of Special Education* **24** (2) 80-87.

Welsh Assembly Government (2006) *Routes for learning: Assessment materials for learners with profound learning difficulties and additional disabilities*. Cardiff: Welsh Assembly Government.

Wigham S & Emerson E (2015) Trauma and life events in adults with intellectual disability. *Current Developmental Disorders Reports* volume 2, 93–99.

Wolfensberger W (1972) *The Principle of Normalisation in Human Services*. Toronto: National Institute on Mental Retardation.

Wolfensberger W (1983) Social role valorisation: A proposed new term for the principle of normalisation. *Mental Retardation* **21** (6) 234–239.

Young H (2016) Conceptualising bereavement in profound and multiple learning disabilities. *Tizard Learning Disability Review* **21** (4) 186–198.

Zeedyk S, Davies C, Parry S & Caldwell P (2009) Fostering social engagement in Romanian children with communicative impairments: The experiences of newly trained practitioners of Intensive Interaction. *British Journal of Learning Disabilities* **37** (3) 186–196.

Zeedyk S, Caldwell P & Davies CE (2009) How rapidly does Intensive Interaction promote social engagement for adults with profound learning disabilities? *European Journal of Special Needs Education* **24** 119–137.

Chapter 10: Adapting dyadic developmental psychotherapy (DDP) to support adults with an intellectual disability who experience complex developmental trauma

Nic Jones

This chapter introduces dyadic developmental psychotherapy (DDP), which the author considers to have more potential to address complex or developmental trauma issues in clinical work with people who have intellectual disabilities (ID). The principles and methods of the approach are explained from the perspective of a clinical psychologist in the National Health Service.

Why DDP?

My work in the field of attachment trauma or developmental trauma has, like my colleagues and likely for you as the reader, been constant throughout my career. However, it took me a while to realise how important and helpful it can be to explicitly make sense of the impact of very early trauma on later development to affect clinical outcomes. I first learned about DDP from my supervisor, Dr Viv Norris, who was helping me with some work that was particularly challenging with an adopted teenager and her family. I noticed my more usual systemic-informed and cognitive-behavioural approaches were not really making a great impact. With her support, I undertook Level 1 DDP training, and then Level 2 the following year – both run by Dan Hughes, who originated this approach. During Level 1 training, I was inspired and encouraged to incorporate this approach with adults with ID. From this point on, my DDP training and supervision would be dual-focused: to include both child and adult ID based work.

Using DDP with people with an ID

My first formal exploration of DDP into my adult-focused work was with two people I'd worked with for some time. Both had originally been referred for individual therapy because the professionals trying to safeguard them were extremely worried and were trying to get the right professionals in place around the clients (one in her early twenties, the other in her late twenties). At the time of referral, both clients were experiencing different but highly chaotic lives. There was a lot of police and statutory service involvement, either because of stealing, physical assault, coercive control by others (at the time this would be referred to as emotional exploitation), high risks of rape, and actual rape, risks of trafficking, high levels of substance misuse, and concerns about financial and emotional exploitation from partners, family and friends. Both had very complicated family relationships, were socially isolated and the services around them were noticing they were often drawn into crisis response for both clients. Both lived in their own premises and were offered community-based support (workers would call to their homes at planned times to assist with shopping, household management etc, depending on their plan of support).

A huge range of services were involved at various points of the clients lives, including the police, GP services, minor injuries unit, midwifery, primary care and secondary care ID, and mental health services. Also, teams within the local authority (housing, disability social workers, safeguarding, children's social workers, leaving care social workers, legal services and the finance department) as well as a number of non-statutory services were involved, which provided various key support (for housing, Women's Aid, Mind). If this feels like a familiar pattern you will know that there were regular professional or network meetings, lots of offers of support and many meetings the clients didn't manage to make. We noticed how for one client there was a noticeable reduction in the number of teams involved when they moved into a house supported by staff that was incorporating a Playful, Accepting, Curious and Empathetic (PACE) approach into their support. PACE is used throughout DDP work and I explore these DDP principles below. Sadly, sometimes, access to supported housing is either declined by the client or we find they do not meet eligibility criteria and so cannot be offered this safety. The containing impact of being able to access immediate safe support fits intrinsically within an attachment-informed approach, illustrated by Golding's House Model of Parenting (2008). Moving into supportive accommodation can be particularly challenging (and, at times, highly resisted) by those whose early experience of care is that it increases risk, reduces safety. Someone with insecure attachments (whether disorganised, ambivalent or avoidant) have learned to manage relationships in order to help them cope or even survive. Moving toward intimacy and care would be counterintuitive to their internal working model of safety. So, while moving into supportive accommodation can dramatically reduce the demands on other services, the impact on the staff teams can be profound, as their role includes not just offering safe support but helping someone adjust to safe care, connection, intersubjective experiences, sharing, taking turns and often a huge loss of power/freedom.

I will focus on working with people living in the community settings but am aware that inpatient settings are noticing the positive impact of DDP to assist within institutional settings.

When I introduced DDP to the two people described above, I had already worked with them for some time – offering them different models of support depending on the presenting issues and what the system or clients needed to prioritise. Both clients were finding it hard to accept the input and guidance from the teams offering them support and help, and we noticed how positive behaviour support (PBS) input and extensive work by hugely experienced professionals was not increasing the safety for these adults at risk. In my therapy work, I had offered a wide range of approaches within the PBS pathway in offering consultation and support to the teams. I had also provided individual therapy (anxiety management, anger management, cognitive behavioural therapy, and eye movement desensitisation and reprocessing (EMDR)), but had to agree with my clients that their distress had not improved. Reflection on the poor progress led me to doubt my clinical skills. Therefore, I talked to both my clients and the teams around them about a DDP model to see if all would be willing to try another, unexplored, approach with me. Thankfully all endorsed trying something new. While change was not immediate, improvements appeared over time. These and other clients have said that they want this information shared, in order to help others. With one client, we actually noticed changes over the years of work via increases in intellectual assessment scores, to the point where they were no longer formally reaching ID criteria. Clients have also welcomed the coherence that PACE provides. Sometimes within DDP we can only focus on the current relationships, but, when offered, it is an approach that can help to make sense of someone's history, emotional experiences, and emotional reactions to others. They can develop an understanding of why it has been profoundly hard to trust, or feel relaxed, and why they previously felt depressed or withdrawn. Finally, they can experience a better sense of connection to others, rather than isolation. I am grateful for my clients' courage and confidence to stick with our therapeutic relationship, and be able to be clear with me about what is and isn't helpful.

What is DDP?

For a full explanation of the theory, practice and empirical basis of DDP please see Hughes *et al.* (2015). I have tried to illustrate how it may work with adults who have ID. Please also see https://ddpnetwork.org.

DDP is a family-based developmental trauma-focused therapy with attachment theory at its core. It uses the principles of PACE to help guide or inform interactions. Ideally, the therapy includes key attachment figures (a current caregiver) in the therapy work and recognises the vital importance of including a person's social network. In children's services, key attachment figure(s), often the parents, are an integral part of the therapy meetings with the aim of helping the child feel safe and regulated (by offering co-regulation), so that they can make sense of their experiences. This work is undertaken alongside their parents, who learn about attachment-focused support in order to either create or deepen the feelings of safety. Strengthening the dyad at home is a goal, rather than focusing on the safety created in the client-therapist relationship alone. In ID work the key attachment figure may well be a paid care-staff team member, taking the role of the safe attachment figure for the person with the attachment-trauma focused issues.

The principles of PACE

PACE stands for an approach that can be:

- **Playful** recognising the need for lighter moments, change of tone or prosody in the voice. There is a clear acknowledgement that we connect when there are moments of fun and delight in each other, and the aim of DDP is to help an insecure person to feel safe.

- **Accepting** another person's experience. While, as professionals, we often feel we endorse or champion a client's viewpoint, sometimes we move quickly on to solutions and ideas for making things better. While it is important to think about strategies at some point, to teach skills, or to challenge underlying beliefs, these approaches can fail to foreground the other person's affective and interpersonal experience. Accepting and hearing about someone's sadness, their anger towards you, or exploring someone's sense of loss can be very difficult, but this acceptance is the starting point for creating coherence for the client; either by validating their experience, or helping them to make sense of their reactions or feelings.

■ **Curious** about another person's experience. Sometimes it is hard to find the right words, or a client might not be able to express their opinions after years of being invalidated or undermined. DDP helps someone notice or consider, with them, what their experience might be like. This needs to be undertaken slowly and sensitively, and, when done at the right pace and in a way that works for the person accessing therapy, can offer a deep sense of coherence about their responses, their reactions, their lived experience. It will likely involve wondering aloud and focusing on affective experiences, rather than a factual account about events.

■ **Empathetic** in orientation. Many therapeutic approaches are deeply empathetic, so this is not unique to DDP. However, when combined with the other aspects of PACE, it creates a powerful way of communicating a deep interest in knowing, making sense, working alongside the client in order to support them. Deep empathy and connection with another increases a sense of being understood or known, which in turn creates a sense of safety through relationships. The focus is on the relationship rather than the behaviour, and can offer opportunities for re-parenting and the neural repair that can follow from a deep sense of safety and connection. In line with Maslow's hierarchy of needs, it could be framed as getting the basics in place first before we consider cognitive, solution-focused or even behavioural change. By creating safety, in allowing someone to potentially experience deeper connection, this can enable significant change in behavioural responses as behaviour is often the expression of distress or dysregulation in the first place.

How DDP impacts on relationships

When supporting adults who have experienced early and significant gaps or failures in care, it can be very helpful to consider how those privations are likely to be impacting on their current experiences, and why non-developmental approaches are inappropriate for these people, at least initially. Repeated experience of poor or frightening care informs our attachment patterns, and like the wording in Brighton rock, our attachment responses become etched into our systems (Bomba 2004, Baylin and Hughes 2016). DDP helps the individual, and crucially those supporting the individual, to make better sense of what their reactions are about and why they respond in the way they do. It can also help members of staff supporting a client to better understand reactions and therefore how to respond in the moment. While using a DDP talking approach there is great use and emphasis on tonality, prosody and proximity (physical and emotional) to each other. Changes in facial features and body gestures are central in our communication, and better support someone with an ID who faces cognitive, social and emotional challenges.

Attuned care and co-regulation

When using a PACE-informed approach, we notice the impact of stepping in to soothe/settle or regulate someone's experience and making a true connection to the other. Attunement refers to our social behaviours where the caregiver, or therapist, looks at the person, notices, and responds often by mirroring the person's facial expression, vocalising their noticing, and responding with a timely to-and-fro. This attunement to another person's experience where there is no attempt to fix, resolve, sort or problem-solve, is felt as a profound form of support, and this is vital for building trust, relationship development and developing empathy for the self. Note that the repair can be both interpersonal and internal. DDP takes a non-evaluative approach and is likely to be a huge shift in experience for people with an ID who can experience daily judgement. DDP discourages the use of more evaluative or even pejorative terms such as 'playing up', 'acting out', 'attention-seeking', 'bad behaviour' or just 'behaviours' to describe distress or changes in response. In particular, the use of 'having a behaviour', as though all we are interested in is problematic social acts or pure functional aspects of our expression, is particularly discouraged, lacking as it is in empathy, playfulness, and acceptance. Curiosity is not enough on its own.

People with ID experience frequent discrimination and potential critique or evaluation possibly as early on as young children, then potentially at school, then later in attempts to access vocational occupation, or in the approaches professionals use in their homes. There is no doubt that working alongside someone and offering such attuned support can be challenging, and in the context of outcome focused and manualised service pathways, it takes great confidence and management support for clinicians to take this time to let a client know you are there while they are upset, angry and frustrated. Focusing work on behaviour change might distract us from offering companionship and support during distress, or encourage us to 'anaesthetise' difficult feelings, or risk-manage signs of anger by encouraging our clients to take time out to 'calm down' on the basis of the time-intensity model of arousal, which suggests that anger will dissipate naturally over time. While in some situations, increasing space can be helpful, so too is the message of benign presence during the tougher times. A sense of unbreakable presence of an attachment figure who will never let us down might be hard to attain, but, when attained, there is very little pain that cannot be endured. This goes for all of us, but especially for those who have not had this gift as children. 'Being there for someone' can sound like a trite soundbite, a cliché, but it is noticeably missing when one looks at cases of people with long-standing trauma. It may be sitting next to someone, moving within someone's eyeline, or playing an instrument, or noisily baking; being available is the key.

Those who were inadvertently 'taught', or who learned to avoid because of consistent parental rebuffing or inconsistent care, will struggle to show their distress directly, and may not have words or a framework for their own big feelings, as no one took the time to reassure, comfort and help them find meaning in their distress. Co-regulation of affect involves creating the safety to make sense (words to describe, symbols for) what is happening so that the experience becomes coherent. Together, in safety, you are piecing together all the factual events and affective changes for someone who is not sure what happened to them. This needs to be done from the client's perspective and it isn't a short process. Lists of challenges and failures – all the things you've done 'wrong' – would switch anyone's attention off and reduces the sense of safety. Instead, by offering deep curiosity about what's happened, we can help reduce a sense of negative or positive evaluation. Acceptance of another's experience and feelings, not rushing to fix or find positive connotation in current responses, even if to the therapist's mind these are problematic, can really help to build the alliance and be the base for establishing trust. Sometimes we may try to reason: 'How do you think so-and-so felt when this happened?' However, this conversation might be lost if the individual has not yet learned empathy for themselves, let alone others. PACE encourages the attachment figures to work alongside the client to find explanations for things that have happened and even if some words are missed, the tone of the voice, the thoughtfulness in the eyes, the gentle nature of our care is how we convey this message. This must be attuned to the client's needs in the same way we can share our concern and love for those who speak a different language or with young babies who have not yet developed speech. It follows that the client communicating primarily by verbal means is not a requirement for DDP, as it derives from those helpful approaches or behaviours shown by emotionally competent parents to their infant. Being alongside another, creating a coherent narrative about the events or the client's feelings, allows the client to trust those around them. It enables co-regulation so that the attachment figures can create practical and emotional safety. Once someone feels better understood and more regulated, they can then reflect on and maybe cope with gentle challenges about the events: the importance of 'Connect before Correct' (Hughes, Golding and Hudson, 2019) is vital.

Dysregulated responses and dissociation, and windows of tolerance

Sometimes a person's reaction to an event can seem disproportionate or unusual given our understanding of the perceived trigger. We notice some people tend to be highly responsive (hyper aroused) in response to stress, while others might become quieter and withdraw (hypo aroused). Someone with an attachment or developmental trauma background will typically live a less-regulated emotional life, and more often experience dysregulation than those with a non-trauma background. There is often a very slim range that a person can operate in, in which they feel OK. The aim of attachment-focused therapy such as DDP is to help broaden the window of tolerance (Siegel, 2012), depicted in Figure 10.1, and, over time, increase their resilience. The highs and lows of such cycles maps on to the internal fluctuations that occur when someone is experiencing extreme distress especially when the reaction seems disproportionate. At the peaks and troughs an individual is no longer regulated and would be described as dysregulated.

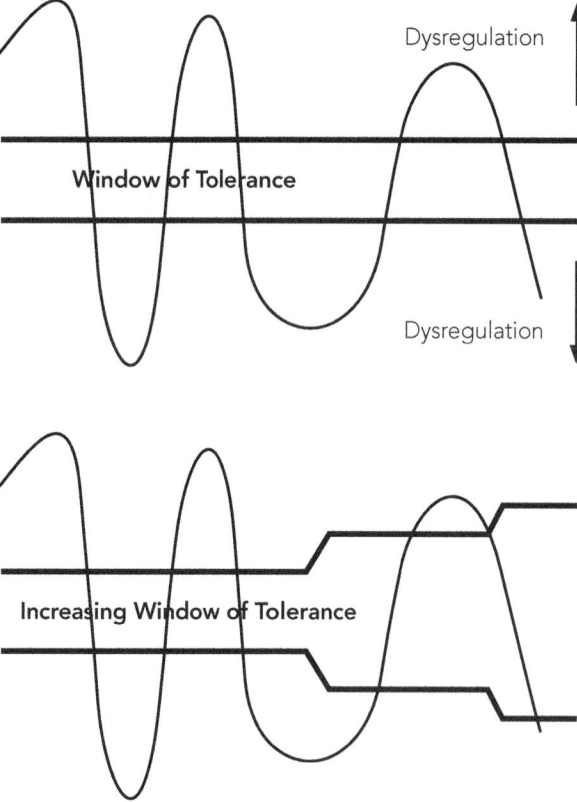

Figure 10.1: Window of tolerance

Someone with an attachment-trauma background is likely to have a very narrow window of tolerance, and the work of Porges (2011) and Dana (2019) has helped us understand regulation is a whole-body experience based on our parasympathetic and sympathetic nervous system. When they are dysregulated or dissociated, a person's reaction might seem bizarre (e.g. they run off when happy; hide in a corner unable to speak, shout manically, etc) and might even be judged to be about an underlying medical condition, such as seizures. Some people are so overwhelmed they might dissociate, resulting in having no memory of the events, which can be very frightening. Safety is central here and the key to increasing regulation is connection (Schore, 2009). It can be helpful and highly empowering for all to test or practise a few regulating activities that can be drawn on in such times of need. DDP works well here alongside other approaches and it can be helpful to include sensory regulation approaches, EMDR, or intensive interaction as appropriate and if already prepared. At all times, the regulatory needs of the person in distress should be central, whether that's about being very high in mood or inactivate or low in affective state.

Primary intersubjective relationships

DDP offers regulation through connection and with the use of the relationship. In connecting with another, we will be impacted by them – this is intersubjective connection (Trevarthen, 2001). This type of connection describes times when what each other does influences the other's experience, and in order to truly connect with another's experience we have to allow ourselves to be impacted. Attachment-trauma repair, or neural repair, is more likely where there is an intersubjective connection, which is based on reciprocity in relationship; knowing that we impact on each other, that our actions, moods and words will affect another person. This type of reciprocity in relationships is empowering for someone who may have very restricted experience that their lives, feelings, experiences touch or influence another. Many people with an ID have experienced years of misunderstandings and have had repeated experiences of powerlessness or worse, threat and harm that seem to recur over decades and without effective oversight (see Flynn and Citarella, 2012; CQC, 2019). DDP supports the development of reciprocity, and deepens the relationship between the primary attachment figure and the client. In order to make friends, have a social life, and feel safe beyond our homes, we first need to experience security in our primary intersubjective relationships.

Implementing DDP: including key attachment figures in therapy

DDP champions and makes central the relationship between the client and a safe attachment figure – ideally one(s) who can be available on a regular basis. As therapists, we can offer regular and predictable support to our clients, but we might only be present for a therapy meeting once a day, once a week, once a month etc. This is a significant and helpful challenge as this model was developed with families in mind and the availability of key attachment figures is important. Bowlby's (1951) original theory was developed, in part, from understanding his own gaps in attachment figures in his life and from observations with other families. He considered very carefully about the feedback systems existing between a child and their mother; the need for security in a home and relationship, support with separations and accessibility of a safe attachment figure. It is likely that these gaps still need to be addressed especially for people with ID, who seem to have more problems with attachment (Hamadi and Fletcher, 2019).

The challenge in adult-focused work is to consider how to best offer similar support and to determine if it is feasible. In all the work I've undertaken, it has not been possible or would not be appropriate or safe for a member of the birth family to be brought into therapy work in this way. Where a client is living in a secure and safe home, the client needs to agree about which member of staff they would like to include in their sessions. When this is difficult to determine, it would be good to consider the key worker, who is likely to have a good knowledge of the client's issues and history. The identified attachment figures or key workers then need to have access to training and guidance about developmental trauma and DDP, to be supported during the therapy with issues that arise, to ideally be allowed to join all the therapy meetings and for their managers to support the therapeutic shift into a deeper intersubjective relationship.

This is understandably a complex and challenging commitment for a care team, and one not without risks as staff do change jobs, can become ill, and need paternity or maternity leave, etc. There are scheduling complications, such as holidays, and an imbalance can emerge as one or two members of staff might build a deeper connection with the client, and information and ideas might not be transferred to other team members. This can be partly addressed by having a core team, who are explicitly named as those supporting the DDP framework with the person. Others can be seen as supporting the core team.

Implementing DDP: impact of therapy on the attachment figures

In the same way we would with a parent or foster carer in child-focused work, there is a need to look after the member of staff who joins the therapy sessions. Sitting with sadness, not moving to solutions, or hearing the impact of abuse or neglect can be very upsetting. The attachment figures are often central to exploring what is helpful and regulating for a client during difficult conversations in and outside of the therapy meeting. These staff need time and support to be able to review actions taken, but also the emotional impact of such connected work.

Implementing DDP: management support and the team around the adult

While a key worker or two might have been identified to join the therapy sessions, it is also important that this is a whole-staff team approach, and the training and teaching about developmental trauma is accessible to all in the immediate staff team. I have found it essential for other professionals in the broader network to access this training to help provide a consistent framework and a shared understanding about the therapeutic work. Often, we need to provide regular consultation meetings for the house staff team to share ideas, have time to make sense of what a client's responses might be about and whether these might link with their developmental trauma or attachment patterns. It can be a chance, if the client agrees, to share issues that are emerging in therapy. Confidentiality is essential and, clearly, we can only discuss what the client feels comfortable sharing.

Sometimes it will not be possible to identify a member of staff to join in therapy, and, where a dyadic approach is not feasible the therapist's focus will turn to the immediate network around the client. With or without a member of staff joining therapy sessions, it is important this work is not undertaken in isolation and the shift to a developmental trauma-informed approach is best developed through whole-team agreements. Parry and Jenkins (2006) outlined the increasingly familiar network training approach, and I have found they can be a helpful step to reviewing existing work, reconsidering formulations (the proposed mechanism maintaining distress or the gap in a relationship change), reviewing risk-management strategies, and allowing time for introductory attachment-focused training. For teams who are familiar with a PBS model, it can be helpful to set aside an additional day to help consider attachment-focused approaches within this framework, how these can sit alongside each other and when attachment focused work is needed before more widely established approaches (See Chapter 8 for more details). This can be a radical shift in some services: sometimes requiring not just multi-agency endorsement but also service commissioners and senior managers to support this as an innovative way of working. It can be costly to involve a member of staff in a therapy session. However, the benefits are considerable and need to be balanced against the huge impact (emotional and also financial) of supporting staff to cope with the distress of ongoing and repeated experiences of behaviours that are of concern, and that can be highly challenging and increase the risk of staff burn-out. On the other hand, when a person is repeatedly presenting with distress and is not responding to other approaches, the healthcare organisation may want to help innovative approaches to address this.

This therapy is focusing on changing relationships; remapping old paradigms or changing what a person does to make themselves feel safer or more regulated, and takes considerable time. In adult work, we are essentially thinking about changing very long-established ways of relating to the world. Yet, by increasing safety and reducing our client's distress, we will be better able to care for our staff, reduce the risks they might experience from behaviours of concern, and increase job or role satisfaction, which, in turn, affects both recruitment and retention.

Blocked care

The work of Hughes and Baylin (2012) addressing 'blocked care' has been significant in helping us make sense of the risks staff face when supporting vulnerable and distressed clients with attachment or developmental trauma. Blocked care occurs when caregivers face stressful circumstances that block any shared enjoyment with the person, and therefore don't get the biological rush that reinforces their empathic response. They may not even seek to be in the same room as the person they are supposed to be caring for, or they notice they feel more critical or at risk of feeling manipulated by a vulnerable client.

We have seen too often, in too many reports, how vulnerable adults in institutional care have been hurt, dehumanised and neglected by those whose job it was to treat, support, nurture and protect from harm, as non-therapeutic services degenerate into mirrored anger, punitive methods, control and restraint (CQC, 2020). DDP can be part of the answer in helping us to understand, undermine and diminish patterns of mutual hostility where large power differentials between the abusers and the abused are repeated.

Hughes and Baylin (2012) described the neurochemical exchanges that we experience in our interactions, what draws us toward another individual and what patterns make us turn away from or, worse, stop caring about someone. It has been hugely powerful to be able to help staff teams understand their different reactions to a person, to make sense of their experiences and to identify whether they are experiencing blocked care. This exploration, based on neurochemical reactions to highly challenging situations and stressors, helps facilitate a non-judgemental exploration of professionals' reactions to their own emotional response to client difficulties. Allowing the discussion enables the difficult issues to be aired, which ultimately means staff can access support and additional supervision and training if and as needed. It also deepens our understanding about the attachment patterns that are triggered in different settings and in different contexts. Someone in blocked care might be able to continue to give practical care, go through the functions of the shift and do all that is required, but they may experience no joy or connection with the client, or, worse, they may become resentful or, in extreme cases, punitive. Sometimes these blocks are there at the start of working together or they can emerge over time. The gaps in connection can arise because repeated rejection and miscuing or challenging behaviours are really wearing. Our brains are switched into connecting with someone (at a neurochemical level) when it feels safe to approach the other person; when there are moments of shared joy and experience; when we feel effective; when we feel we can make sense of and empathise with the other; and when we can make sense of why the last shift was so hard for everyone. This is the same for staff and clients alike. This is a feedback loop – our connections with each other feel good or inadequate because of what Baylin and Hughes (2012) suggest are at the neurochemical level releases of oxytocin and dopamine (attachment/love and reward systems). Our interpretation of events, ability to make sense of a difficult day and access to supervision to support these reflections can therefore be pivotal in determining our relationships. Helping a staff team to understand that their responses and some of the more difficult feelings make sense is vital. It helps provide a framework for discussion and ongoing support with the aim of reducing and better managing risks.

Safety plans

I have found it helpful in most of my work with clients to ask them to create a safety plan with me. I have adapted an outline from Kim Golding and found a picture-based summary to be very empowering and helpful, to both consolidate what we are noticing in therapy, but also as a reminder about what the client and others can do when they notice signs of dysregulation. This model is no doubt similar to other risk-management summaries, but my clients have found it very useful. This makes me keen to include it in this summary – it can, of course, be a word- or video-recorded summary; using the best medium for the client is vital.

Figure 10.2 is a variation on the safety plan originally outlined by Kim Golding (2008), adapted in turn from Sprague (1997), Clinical management of suicidal behaviour in children and adolescents, Sage Publications.

Figure 10.2: Safety plan

My name is
A bit about me: my hopes and dreams, things I like about myself and things that are more difficult about myself.

I love my friends and family

I need to talk when I'm worried

I find it hard to say what's feeling bad

I get upset and depressed when I'm ill

Why I feel I need a reminder plan?

When I am very upset, I may cry and once I hurt myself

I want to have a plan everyone knows about

Things that worry me

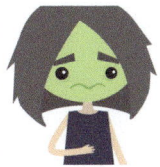 When I'm very ill and
don't know why

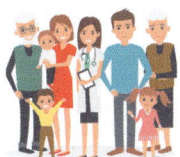 My family's health

Signs that I am worried in my body

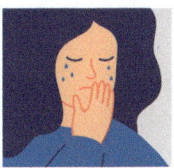 Crying

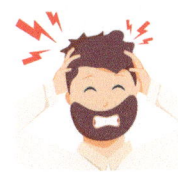 Headache

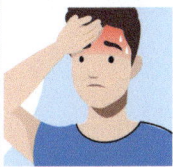 Sweating

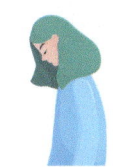 Feel sad/depressed

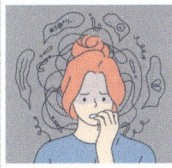 Blame myself for stuff

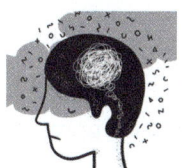 Call myself bad names

What helps?

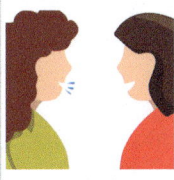 Talking

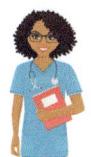 Check my health with GP

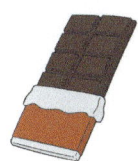 Chocolate

How can others help me?

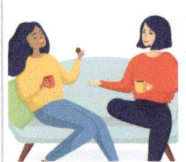
Get out of the house – visit a friend

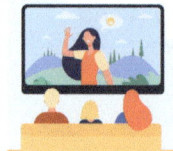
Watch TV with me

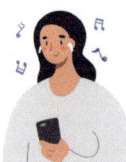
Listen to music and dance with me

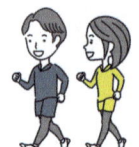
See if someone will go for a walk

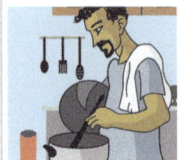
Cook a meal

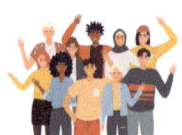
Go to the group

Qualifications and working within the model

DDP overlaps with many other approaches and the outline of PACE sounds similar to other approaches, but all practitioners who use this approach note how challenging it is. It is strongly advised to attend DDP Level 1 training before considering offering any therapeutic work using PACE or PACE informed approaches, and regular DDP supervision is also considered essential to ensure good practice is maintained.

References

Bowlby J (1951) Maternal care and mental health. *Bulletin of the World Health Organization* **3** 355–533.

Dana D (2018) *The Polyvagal Theory in Therapy*. London: Norton

Bomba J (2004) Attachment and brain development. *Przeglad lekarski* **61** (11) 1272–4.

CQC (2019) *Cygnet Whorlton Hall new approach comprehensive report Independent Health Care* [online] – MH Location Jul 2019 Cygnet Whorlton Hall New Approach Comprehensive Report (IndependentHealthCare-MH Location Jul 2019)_INS2-6853743651 (cqc.org.uk)

CQC (2020) *Out of sight – who cares? A review of restraint, seclusion and segregation for autistic people and people with a learning disability and/or mental health condition*. Care Quality Commission, October 2020.

Flynn M & Citarella V (2012) *Winterbourne View Hospital: A serious case review*. UK: South Gloucestershire Council publication.

Golding K (2008) *Nurturing Attachments: Supporting children who are fostered or adopted*. London: JKP.

Hamadi L & Fletcher HK (2019) Are people with an intellectual disability at increased risk of attachment difficulties? A critical review. *Journal of Intellectual Disabilities*. July 30

Hughes D, Golding KS & Hudson J (2015) Dyadic developmental psychotherapy (DDP): The development of the theory, practice and research base. *Adoption & Fostering* **39** (4) 356-365.

Hughes DA and Baylin J (2012) *Brain-based Parenting: The neuroscience of caregiving for health attachment*. London: Norton.

Hughes DA, Golding KS & Hudson J (2019) *Healing Relational Trauma with Attachment-focused Interventions*. London: Norton.

Jenkins R & Parry R (2006) Working with the support network: Applying systemic practice in learning disabilities services. *British Journal of Learning Disabilities* **34** (2) 77–81.

Porges SW (2011) *The Polyvagal Theory: Neuropsychological foundations of emotions, attachment, communication, self-regulation*. London: Norton.

Schore AN (2009) *Attachment trauma and the developing right brain. Origins of disorders: DSM-V and beyond*. London: Routledge.

Siegel D (2012) *The Developing Mind: How relationships and the brain interact to shape who we are*. London: The Guilford Press.

Trevarthen C (2001) Intrinsic motives for companionship in understanding: Their origin, development, and significance for infant mental health. *Infant Mental Health Journal* **22** (1-2) 95-131.

Chapter 11: Trauma-informed psychodynamic psychotherapy

Nigel Beail

Psychodynamic psychotherapy has developed from psychoanalysis. Psychoanalysis and its derivatives – psychoanalytic and psychodynamic psychotherapy – were considered to be unsuitable therapies for people who have intellectual disabilities (ID) until this was challenged in the 1980s. Psychoanalysis, being five times a week, is expensive to deliver, not widely available and has only had a limited application with people who have ID (De Groef and Heinemann 1999; Shepherd and Beail, 2017). However, since the 1980s, psychodynamic psychotherapy has been adapted and made accessible for people who have ID (Beail, 2016; Beail and Jackson, 2013; Frankish, 2016; Jackson and Beail, 2013). Psychodynamic psychotherapy has a little more flexibility, is delivered less frequently and can be time-limited like other psychological interventions available today. The approach described here is based on the model outlined by Malan (2001) in the form of two triangles (see figure 11.1).

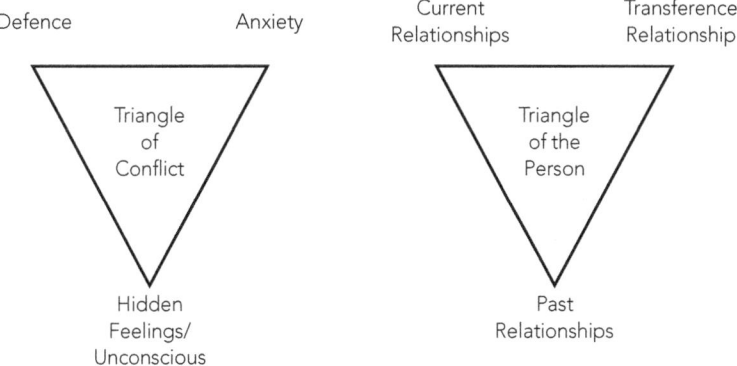

Figure 11.1: Malan's triangles of conflict and the person (2001)

The triangle of conflict is used to help the person process emotional experiences that are outside of conscious awareness. This contains unconscious memories and impulses (hidden), emotional experience (anxiety), and the way the person prevents these from becoming conscious (defence). This is an interpersonal or relational approach and so attempts to help the person understand how their difficulties as represented in the triangle of conflict are active in the three corners of the triangle of the person. So, for example, the defences used to ward off anxiety and keep feelings out of conscious thought in the person's current interpersonal relationships will have developed in their past relationships. These will then manifest in the relationship with the therapist (transference in the triangle of the person). The therapist is concerned with the defences the person employs (defence) to deal with feelings of anxiety caused by unconscious and past experiences. The approach is time-limited and maintains a therapeutic focus, as opposed to free association as in longer-term psychoanalytic approaches.

It is important for the therapist to have an understanding of the developmental factors that influence an individual's experience of themselves and others from their earliest relationships and attachments onwards. Thus, when a person meets someone for the first time, they will not engage in unique behaviours, but enter the relationship by applying what they have experienced and learned through past relationships in order to make sense of this new situation. So, when a person begins psychotherapy, they enter a new relationship and, in doing so, apply previously formed ways of relating to this new situation. As people enter therapy due to problematic experiences in their relationships, these patterns re-emerge in the relationship with the therapist. Thus, current and past relationship patterns become reactivated and replayed as the problematic experiences the person brings to therapy are explored. Freud called this process transference and the triangle of the person helps the client explore how past issues in relationships can often become a feature of current relationships and then in the relationship with the therapist.

Trauma-informed psychodynamic psychotherapy is informed by Freud's trauma theory as outlined in his paper *The Aetiology of Hysteria* (Freud, 1896). Here, Freud linked traumatic experiences to the development of psychological distress and mental health problems (see chapter 4). The traumas Freud referred to at the time included rape, abuse, and aggression. He described his new psychoanalytic method as leading the patient's attention back from their current presenting problem or symptom as experienced in current relationships with others (current relationships in the triangle of the person) to the scene in which and through which the symptom arose – a scene of significant traumatic force in the past (past in the triangle of the person). He put forward the theory that these traumatic experiences were thrust out of conscious thought into the unconscious (hidden in the triangle of conflict) through the action of a defence mechanism (defence in the triangle of conflict). Freud also described how people presenting with psychological distress do so because a present-day event causes the past traumatic experiences to come into operation in the form of unconscious memories. It is the presence of these unconscious memories that give rise to the symptoms of psychological distress (anxiety in the triangle of conflict). Freud (1896) noted that the problem that led to the person being referred to him bore no relation to the nature of the distress the client presents. The reason for this was that the current presenting events or problem was linked to the now unconscious trauma of the past. Freud claimed his new method of psychoanalysis helps the client on a path back to the memory of the earlier trauma. So, the presenting issues have the significance of a connecting link in the chain of associations to earlier scenes of greater traumatic force. Freud went on to change his theory to one in which the traumas were phantasies. However, his original theory has subsequently been embraced.

Today, trauma-informed psychodynamic psychotherapy embraces the earlier discoveries of Freud (1896), Ferenczi (1932) and Klein (1932) in that the therapists hold in mind that trauma is a possible cause of the psychological distress the clients present with.

To clarify the process that takes place we need to understand Freud's later (1940) model of the mind. Freud described this consisting of three parts: the id; the ego; and the super-ego. Of concern here is the ego, which functions as an intermediary between the unconscious part of the mind (hidden) and the real world where traumas occur (current and past relationships). The ego acts in the service of self-preservation in the form of helping the person to avoid or adapt to situations, or, through activity, bring about changes to their advantage using defence mechanisms such as denial and repression (defence). Over time and through the work of several psychoanalytic practitioners, a wide range of defence mechanisms have been identified, and people who have ID make use of most of them (Newman and Beail, 2010). The ego uses these defence mechanisms to enable the person to put disagreeable things, such as traumatic experiences, out of mind, which may render them unconscious (hidden). Freud also described a further internal agency called the super-ego, into which we take representations of our parents into our self and the parental influence is prolonged. However, before this, Freud (1896) described how traumatic experience can be internalised, which was a forerunner of what became object relations theory, in which a whole range of people with whom we have relationships are internalised.

People come into therapy due to having problematic experiences and feelings of distress. The assimilation of problematic experiences model was developed from research with the general population (Stiles *et al.*, 1990), which showed that most people enter therapy at what they called the 'problem statement' level. Thus, the client could articulate what they thought was their problem. Using this model with people with ID, Newman and Beail (2005) found that they present for treatment at the lower levels of assimilation – such as 'warded off', experiencing 'unwanted thoughts', or having some 'vague awareness' of the problem. However, they also demonstrated that psychodynamic psychotherapy can enable clients with ID to move towards and beyond the level of problem statement in psychodynamic psychotherapy.

When people are referred for help and then present as warded off or as having unwanted thoughts or vague awareness of their problem then the way forward in psychodynamic psychotherapy is to empathically engage with the person and enable an exploration of their difficulties. The initial focus is on current issues in the client's life (current relationships), but with an understanding that these are linked to previous difficulties in their past as reflected in Malan's triangle of the person.

The therapeutic frame

In trauma-informed psychodynamic psychotherapy, the therapist provides one-to-one, weekly sessions preferably in the same private room with comfortable seating where the therapist and client sit at about a 90-degree angle to each other. However, some flexibility around the duration of sessions may be needed as some people may have low tolerance for the usual duration of 50 minutes. Some clients may need the support of someone they know well at first. So, the therapist gives the client time to feel safe with them before asking the supporter to sit in the waiting room. Such a pre-therapy phase needs to be managed well to avoid any threats to confidentiality.

The therapeutic process

The therapist forms a relationship with the client through showing curiosity about them. The therapist uses several ways to help the client to tell their story. The psychodynamic psychotherapist works with the understanding that when they empathically engage with their client – this facilitates transference. The client's internal representations of experiences in current and past relationships can be good and some may be bad, due to links to negative or traumatic experiences involving them. For Freud (1912), transference is defined as when psychological experiences are revived and, instead of being in the past, are applied to dealings with a person in the present. Transference allows the therapist to identify interpersonal issues and deal with them as empirical data in the here-and-now. For example, if the client spends most of their time when with people talking about cars, they are highly likely to do the same with the therapist. The therapist may try and focus on why the client has been referred, but then the client quickly returns to telling them about cars. Thus, by changing the subject (defence), the therapist identifies that the client has something they want to keep out of conscious thought and communication (hidden).

Psychodynamic therapists work has been described as consisting of listening and observing and seeking clarification, using confrontation, and making interpretations (Sublette and Novick, 2004 and illustrated with people who have ID in Beail, 1989). The therapist seeks information from the client seeking responses aimed at clarification, which helps sort out what is happening by questioning and rephrasing. Exploratory responses are generated from hypotheses about what the client might not be saying in words but could be hinting at through behaviour or tone of voice. The therapist may initially reflect to the client what they have said or done in the session. They draw attention to something the client may not mention such as their parents, their disability or other significant relationships. The therapist observes the client's response to this. For example, the therapist's action may raise the client's anxiety and result in the use of a defence mechanism to try to reduce this. This may lead to a gentle confrontation to draw the client's attention to the defence i.e. 'when I said this, you denied it or changed the subject'. The aim of the therapist would be to reduce the defensive inhibition to enable the client to progress to explore their memories, feelings and fantasies. The therapist also focuses on what it is like to be with this person. Thus, the therapist starts to feel what it is like for others to be with this client, which, in psychodynamic psychotherapy, we call the countertransference.

Case material

Simon was referred initially for bereavement issues, difficulties in his current relationships and with a past history of alleged sexually inappropriate behaviour. In his assessment session, he said he had a difficult childhood and had flashbacks. In therapy when I tried to seek information about his childhood and the content of the flashbacks, he told me he felt angry and upset, he became tearful and then changed the subject to talk about something else. In psychodynamic psychotherapy, this is understood as Simon bringing defences into play to ward off the anxiety he felt at the emergence of past memories from his unconscious. The therapist draws the client's attention to what they are doing (reflect back): 'I asked you about your flashbacks, you said you felt sad and angry (past relationships), you then became upset (anxiety).' I then used a gentle confrontation, '...and then you changed the subject (defence)'. Simon did not say anything about the content of the flashbacks. I said this was difficult for him, to think about the past, and that he had not had the opportunity to do so. I explained again the boundaries of therapy in that this was a safe place for him to talk about his feelings and what had happened to him. It gradually emerged that the memories he wished to keep out of conscious communication were of physical violence he received at the hand of his parents.

During this part of the therapeutic process, the psychodynamic psychotherapist will be forming initial hypotheses that would help the client make sense of their problem, but hold them silently while gathering data to support or refute them. For Simon, my initial intervention was to draw his attention to his defence (changing the subject) and link this to his anxiety (being upset in the session) to what he was trying to keep out of conscious thought (violence in past relationships). Thus, the three corners of Malan's (2001) triangle of conflict are linked together. The aim of doing this is to help the client understand these links and work through them to resolve them so they can live with the memories in a less problematic way. For Simon, the process will now involve him gradually feeling enabled to talk about the past traumatic experiences.

Clients who have experienced trauma in their lives may communicate traumatic material in very different ways. James, a young man with ID and autism, was referred due to a severe bereavement reaction. He refused the offer of psychotherapy. However, due to the severity of his problems, we kept in touch with him. It took him about a year to accept the offer of psychotherapy. The early session focused on his bereavement, but James talked about something he had not told anyone before – a series of physical and sexually abusive recollections from his early childhood. The abuse stopped as the perpetrator was caught in the act and James had not seen the perpetrator again. The abuse he described was quite vivid in his mind. Thus, James presented traumatic material very early in his therapy. I began my work with James seeking clarification of his recollections, but this, as it did with Simon, met with resistance in the form of changing the subject. As the work progressed, he started to experience times when he felt the abuser over him and his breath against him. The abuse stopped about 15 years ago and his family, who stopped it, never spoke about this again. James could not speak about it when it happened as the abuse occurred when he had not developed language, and he did not start talking until several years after the abuse ceased. In terms of defences, James had split off and disowned the experience of the abusive relationship but had not been able to repress it all. However, he started to show awareness that he may have put some memories of the abuse completely out of mind through the intrusive thoughts and feeling he experienced. As we explored his development, a story emerged of him trying to keep the abuse out of mind, but this gave rise to a childhood of anger and aggression towards others, which resulted in exclusion from every educational establishment he attended. However, this was not seen at the time as communication of distress, but as difficult behaviour. Now that James could tell his story, the therapist attends to factual content, words used and what is unsaid, clarifying meaning where necessary, through asking open questions.

Therapists need to acknowledge the often-limited expressive communication skills of people with ID, and so multiple modes of communication may be needed. Equal weight needs to be given to non-verbal behaviours, and the use of expressive materials such as paper and pens and representative objects such as figures may assist. Klein (1932) showed us the power of using play as a medium with children. So, the provision of some more age or developmentally appropriate materials can assist adults who have ID to communicate. Tom communicated the problematic experiences in his mind through drawing the people involved in the trauma in a big circle, which he said was his head, on a large sheet of paper. Klein (1932) also observed that some children brought things to sessions that had meaning or a communicative function in relation to their distress. Janet was referred due to her difficulties in relationships with the people she shared a supported home with since a fellow resident had expressed a desire to have a relationship with her. She was becoming at risk of losing her place there. Janet began weekly sessions but struggled to talk about her problems. Then she produced a pen from her pocket and showed it to me. The pen had two men wearing suits on it. She then turned the pen upside-down and this revealed the two men naked. Unsure at this point as to its meaning I reflected back to her what she had done. In the next session, we continued to explore her difficulties in relationships. This time she produced an ethnic doll and placed it on the table. Again, unsure as to its meaning I reflected back what she had done. She then hit the doll on its head and a penis emerged from under its tunic. There was now a theme emerging. In the next session, Janet arrived a few minutes late wearing an apron. She told me she had been making jam tarts. In this session she stood up and raised the apron to reveal a huge pretend penis. There was now a theme; Freud referred to occurrences such as this in the transference as repetition compulsion due to an unconscious memory. Each object, the pen, the doll and the apron were all making fun of the male organ. Thus, Janet was using humour as a defence about her anxieties about the penis. I therefore linked the three acts together and put to her that she was making fun of the penis because she felt anxious about it and the fun reduced her anxiety. This interpretation took her on a gradual road back to her traumatic childhood experiences of being sexually abused in the care system.

Freud (1896) described the process whereby people who have been sexually abused can act out their abuse with others. Klein (1932) similarly described this behaviour in the children she was working with. My client, John, was referred because he was seen to sexually assault a young child in the street. The police were called, and he was taken to the station. There it was decided, due to his ID, he should be diverted from court to treatment. The police informed me that John had previously been abducted, and taken to a remote area and sexually assaulted. During his therapy, John reported recurring traumatic dreams. In the dreams, he was taken away from his siblings. The perpetrator had a gun and he ended up covered in blood. These dreams were found to be remarkably consistent with details given to me by the police at the time of referral; John left his siblings playing to go to the toilet. He was later found by the police in a state of distress and soaked in blood and urine. Examination found he had been seriously sexually assaulted. The dream did not need interpreting as such, but the aspects of the dream needed to be related to what he experienced. This process in therapy led to the dream to not occur again. However, we needed to continue therapy for John to process and work through the extreme abuse he had suffered.

Klein (1932) also described a child acting out sexually in the session with her. People who have IDs who have been the victims of trauma may not have the words to communicate what has happened to them. This is because the iconic system (visual memories) and the symbolic system (language to describe those memories) are dyssynchronous in people who have ID (Beail, 2013). So, the process of empathic engagement and the development of a trusting therapeutic alliance may lead to the client accessing traumatic memories, but being unable to describe or talk about what happened. Thus, they may act out a past traumatic experience in the therapy room or in the transference. Sinason (1992) worked with a boy called Ali who had limited communication and, like James, was violent and disruptive at school. However, unlike James, Ali was referred for therapy, which he started at the age of eight years. After a year of free play, Sinason introduced some new toys into the therapy room. Ali's communication skills were seen to develop and he produced his first grammatically correct sentence. However, the content of what he said was sexual and his actions with the toys was sexual. Thus, applying the concept of transference, Ali was acting out sexual scenes in the session that he had been exposed to. Similarly, Beail and Newman (2005) describe Alan's behaviour in a session. Alan acted out in a sexual way towards the therapist, first by rubbing his legs, then his penis over his trousers and then went to take his penis out. Aggression can also be acted out in the session. Steven was referred for difficulties in his relationship with his mother. He was acting in an aggressive manner towards her. Exploration of his difficulties led to Steven telling me about and describing the beatings he had received from his stepfather. However, I noticed in our exploration that Steven did not mention his own father. When I drew this to his attention, he jumped up with his fists clenched in a threatening manner towards me. Stephen, Ali and Alan were all acting out in the here-and-now/transference corner of Malan's triangle. Perry (1990) defines acting out as a form of defence where the individual deals with emotional conflicts, or internal or external stressors, by acting without reflection or apparent regard for negative consequences. It involves the expression of feelings, wishes and impulses in uncontrolled behaviour with apparent disregard for personal or social consequences. Perry goes on to state that acting out usually occurs in response to interpersonal events with significant people in the person's life. For Steven, Ali and Alan acting out or acting in the session allows for the discharge and expression of feelings and impulses, rather than tolerate them and think about the painful experiences that caused them.

In the therapy sessions, Steven, Ali and Alan all attempted to deal with their sexual or aggressive feelings through the process of projective identification. Projective identification occurs when a current or past relationship is transferred into the relationship with the therapist. Steven, Ali and Alan experienced their feelings as unacceptable and split off and projected these into the therapist, as if it was really the therapist that originated them. For the client, it is now just like being with the person who committed the physical or sexual assault. So, the client behaves towards the therapist as if they are with that person or the therapist is just like that person. Thus, for Steven this was understood as him expecting the therapist to be violent and so he jumped up to defend himself. Ali asked Sinason to suck his penis and Alan started to get his penis out for the therapist. This is understood as them expecting the same response from the therapist as they would their abuser. Such acting out needs to be contained and Alvarez (2012) has recommended a level of interpretation she calls intensified vitalising. Here the therapist basically brings the client back into the room by making a clear call. Alvarez called this 'Hey', but this can be achieved by clearly and firmly saying the person's name and asking them to stop what they are doing. Then the therapist tries to move the client to using more appropriate means of expression. For Alan and Ali this involved helping them develop a vocabulary to describe their feelings and actions, including learning words for body parts and sexual acts.

In summary, in order to understand the hidden (unconscious) feelings, the therapist must identify the defences and the anxiety and draw these to the client's attention. Then they make links between stages of the conflict and between life stages, represented by the second of Malan's triangles, the triangle of the person. This depicts the origin of the information: the setting in therapy (the transference) and a comment might be, 'you feel like this when you are here with me', then to the person's present living environment, 'you feel like this towards your friend', and then the person's past i.e. 'you felt like this towards your abuser' (See Figure 11.1).

Another approach to helping the client make sense of their communication in the transference is to change the location of the feelings from 'you' to 'others'. Alvarez (2012) called this the describe level of interpretation. So, for a client such as Stephen, who is acting in an angry manner towards the therapist, the therapist may extend a reflective comment, 'You feel angry…'. To make an interpretation, we go on to say, 'You feel angry because your father hit you…'. Alvarez called this the explanatory level. However, it may be that the person with ID may not accept an interpretation with this location i.e. 'you' as the 'you' may be felt as nothing but angry, which they find intolerable and so defend against this. So, for example, it may be better to say, 'Part of you feels angry'. However, this may also fail to be accepted and so Alvarez (2012) suggests using the ideas of Winnicott, and locating the feeling, behaviour or issue in others. So, we may say something like: 'Most people find it annoying when people get angry.' However, when the acting out challenges the boundaries of therapy, as Simon's did, the interpretation may have to be put on hold and the therapist need to bring the client back into the reality of the relationship with the therapist, rather than the transferred one they are acting into by gaining the client attention. With Stephen, as with Alan, this was achieved by clearly and firmly saying his name (intensified vitalising).

Conclusion

Trauma-informed psychodynamic psychotherapy offers people who have ID an alternative or preferred approach to the treatment of psychological distress and behavioural difficulties, especially when they present at the lower levels of assimilation of their problematic experience. Psychodynamic psychotherapy can be provided to work alongside other frameworks such as a positive behavioural support plan (Chapter 8). The therapeutic frame is virtually the same as that in general psychodynamic practice but with some flexibility around length of sessions, use of materials in sessions and negotiated involvement of relatives and carers. The approach needs some adaptation to take account of the client's developmental needs and communication abilities. Working with clients who have been traumatised means listening to and working with very difficult material. I have been shocked by the reaction of some people I have taught who have made comments in response to descriptions of sexual acting out, such as 'I should not have to put up with this', or, 'I would leave the room'. Such responses would be anti-therapeutic and not evidence-based. The evidence base is clear that one of the core qualities of an effective therapist is one who holds a strong alliance with the client (Baldwin *et al.*, 2007), does not avoid difficult topics in therapy (Wampold, 2011) and are able to respond to difficult moments during therapy (Anderson *et al.*, 2020). Thus, the trauma-informed psychodynamic psychotherapist needs to be aware of the likelihood of acting out in the session and respond to it effectively in a supportive and containing way.

Evidence is emerging to shows that this approach can be effective (Shepherd and Beail, 2017; Skelly *et al.*, 2017), and that recipients who have ID value it and are satisfied with it (Khan and Beail, 2013; Merriman and Beail, 2009; Statham and Beail, 2018).

References

Alvarez A (2012) *The Thinking Heart: Three levels of psychoanalytic therapy with disturbed children*. London: Routledge.

Anderson T, Finkelstein JD & Horvath SA (2020) The facilitative interpersonal skills method: Difficult psychotherapy moments and appropriate therapist responsiveness. *Counselling and Psychotherapy Research* **20**, 463–469.

Baldwin SA, Wampold BE & Imel, ZE (2007) Untangling the alliance-outcome correlation: Exploring the relative importance of therapist and patient variability in the alliance. *Journal of Consulting and Clinical Psychology* **75**, 842-852.

Beail N (2013) The role of cognitive factors in psychodynamic psychotherapy with people who have intellectual disabilities. *The Psychotherapist* **53** 8-10.

Beail N (2016) Psychodynamic psychotherapy. In: N Beail (Ed) *Psychological Therapies and People who have Intellectual Disabilities* (pp22-27). Leicester: British Psychological Society.

Beail N (2017) Individual psychodynamic psychotherapy. In: J Davies & C Nagi (Eds) *Individual Psychological Therapies in Forensic Settings*. London: Routledge.

Beail N & Jackson T (2013) Psychodynamic psychotherapy and people with intellectual disabilities. In: JL Taylor, WR Lindsay, RP Hastings & C Hatton (Eds) *Psychological Therapies for Adults with Intellectual Disabilities*. Chichester: Wiley.

Beail N & Newman D (2005) Psychodynamic counselling and psychotherapy for mood disorders. In: P Sturmey (Ed) *Mood Disorders in People with Mental Retardation* (pp 273-292). Kingston NY: NADD Press. De Groef J & Heinemann E (1999) Psychoanalysis and Mental Handicap. London, Free Association Books.

Ferenczi S (1932) Confusion of Tongues between adults and the child (New Translation by JM Masson & M Loring 1985) In: JM Mason (1985) *The Assault on Truth: Freud and Child Sexual Abuse* (pp 291-303). London: Fontana.

Frankish P (2016) *Disability Psychotherapy: An innovative approach to trauma-informed care*. London: Karnac.

Freud S (1896) The aetiology of hysteria. *The Standard Edition of the Complete Psychological Works of Sigmund Freud* (3 pp191–221). London: Hogarth.

Freud S (1912) The dynamics of transference. *The Standard Edition of the Complete Psychological Works of Sigmund Freud* (12, pp 97–108). London: Hogarth.

Freud S (1940) An outline of psychoanalysis. *The Standard Edition of the Complete Psychological Works of Sigmund Freud* (Vol. 23). London: Hogarth.

Jackson T & Beail N (2013) The practice of individual psychodynamic psychotherapy with people who have intellectual disabilities. *Psychoanalytic Psychotherapy* **27**, 108-123.

Khan M & Beail N (2013) Service user satisfaction with individual psychotherapy for people who have intellectual disabilities. *Advances in mental health and Intellectual Disabilities* **7**, 277–283.

Klein M (1932) *The Psychoanalysis of Children*. London: Hogarth Press.

Malan DH (2001) *Individual Psychotherapy and The Science of Psychodynamics*. London: Butterworth.

Merriman C & Beail N (2009) Service user views of long-term individual psychodynamic psychotherapy. *Advances in Mental Health and Learning Disabilities* **3** 42–47.

Newman DW & Beail N (2005) An analysis of assimilation during psychotherapy with people who have mental retardation. *American Journal on Mental Retardation* **110**, 359–365.

Newman DW & Beail N (2010) An exploratory study of the defence mechanisms used in psychotherapy by adults who have intellectual disabilities. *Journal of Intellectual Disability Research* **54**, 579–583.

Perry CJ (1990) *Defence mechanisms Rating Scales*. Cambridge, MA: Cambridge Hospital.

Shepherd C & Beail N (2017) A systematic review of the effectiveness of psychoanalysis, psychoanalytic and psychodynamic psychotherapy with adults with intellectual disability: Progress and challenges. *Psychoanalytic Psychotherapy* **31** 94–117.

Sinason V (1992) *Mental Handicap and the Human Condition: New approaches from the Tavistock*. London: Free Association Books.

Skelly A, McGeehan C & Usher R (2018) An open trial of psychodynamic psychotherapy with people who have mild-moderate intellectual disabilities with waiting list and follow up controls. *Advances in Mental Health and Intellectual Disabilities* **12** (5-6) 153–162.

Statham V & Beail N (2018) Service user views on the acceptability, accessibility and effectiveness of psychodynamic psychotherapy. *International Journal of Developmental Disabilities* **64** 175–183.

Stiles WB, Elliott R, Llewelyn SP, Firth-Cozens JA, Margison FR Shapiro DA & Hardy GE (1990) Assimilation of problematic experiences by clients in psychotherapy. *Psychotherapy* **27** 411–420.

Sublette M E & Novick J (2004) Essential techniques for the beginning psychodynamic psychotherapist. *American Journal of Psychotherapy* **58** (1) 67–75.

Wampold,BE (2011). Qualities and actions of effective therapists. *American Psychological Association* [online]. Available at: http://www.apa.org/education/ce/effective-therapists.pdf.

Chapter 12: Interventions based on the Mahler model of emotional development

Pat Frankish

After completing an assessment of the emotional developmental stage of an individual showing signs of attachment and delayed emotional difficulties, the next question that arises is: 'How do we use this information to design and deliver an intervention that will facilitate further development?' Probably the most exciting part of my work developing an assessment tool (Frankish, 2019), was discovering that the condition of arrested development is not static but can be ameliorated. Having for many years been told that people cannot change because of their intellectual disability (ID), it was very gratifying to realise that they can. But this is dependent upon the recognition and acceptance of the cause of the developmental delay. Once it has become clear that an individual can be 25-years-old physically, six-years-old cognitively, but 18-months-old emotionally, it becomes possible to plan an intervention that meets their emotional needs. What has also become apparent from using the emotional development model described in Chapter 5, is that facilitating progress in the emotional development allows for more flexibility in the cognitive area. This can, of course, be linked to what we know about anxiety, which hinders the availability of cognitive functioning.

Mahler

In Mahler's model, she has six stages, while the Frankish assessment of the impact of trauma (Frankish, 2019) just uses four stages. This is because the first stage of symbiosis and the sixth stage of individuation is very rarely seen in practice. So, the four stages of differentiation, practising, early rapprochement, and late rapprochement are the ones that are used and referred to in this chapter. However, it is worth mentioning that if working with a newborn who is struggling to establish a symbiotic relationship with its mother or primary carer, then referral to Mahler's symbiotic stage would be a good idea. It is also worth noting that people who have reached individuation but may have suffered trauma after that, will need a different approach more akin to trauma-informed psychological therapy.

Differentiation

If we assess someone as being stuck at the differentiation stage they will be significantly cut off from the world and most, if not all, of their behaviours will be self-referenced. They will have very little connection with anyone, and will seek only to have a relief of physical issues such as hunger, cold, toilet needs and such like. This is the range of behaviours that would be found in a very young baby up to a few months old. The parental role at that stage is to keep the baby safe, warm, fed, and it would be pointless to expect the baby to do anything in exchange for the services provided. However, an adult who is stuck at this emotional developmental stage will usually be expected to interact with staff or family. They are, of course, unable to express gratitude for anything that is provided for them and this is one of the aspects that leads to their paucity of emotional support. A programme of intervention for someone stuck at this stage would involve giving attention and affection, with eye contact, if it can be tolerated by the individual, at regular intervals. If a programme of contact every 20 minutes or half an hour is put in place, then within a few weeks the individual will start looking for the approach from the member of staff. And once they start to look for you coming, you can make a connection and facilitate further growth. It can feel quite hard to do this at first, but it gets easier as time goes on. Emotional warmth and asking nothing in return is what is required, so it is important not to ask a question, even if it is 'How are you', as the individual is not able to answer the question, and there is an increase in tension, and they withdraw. Asking how somebody is is usually seen as a positive thing to do, so it takes a bit of practice to go up to someone and say 'Hi, I have come to see you and I brought you a drink', instead of 'Would you like a drink?' but, with practice, it gets easier and it is effective.

Most of the people who are stuck at the differentiation stage will be people with profound disabilities or severe autism. They will have suffered trauma in the first few weeks and months of life, possibly in intensive care, or with feeding difficulties. There is insufficient support for new mothers who struggle to feed their babies. And the babies do not choose to be difficult to feed. There is usually a reason, but it may be some time before it is sorted out, and this tiny baby may become traumatised by the pain of being hungry. And sometimes they shut down. This may or may not be noticed depending on their other skills. So, if they develop normally physically and cognitively, it may not be noticed that they are emotionally shut down, and they may very quickly get a diagnosis of autism. By this time, they will be likely to be autistic because the brain will not have developed its emotional capacity.

Once the person has responded to the contact, it is possible to introduce activities which turn very quickly into practising behaviours. These are repetitive and skill-based, so it is very important to offer opportunities to succeed.

Practising

If the initial assessment indicates that the stuck stage is practising, then we are looking at behaviours equivalent to the ten- to 15-month-old child. This is still a stage where the expectation is to receive attention, support and care without having to provide anything in return. So again, there is no gratitude shown towards staff or family, no ability to recognise the needs or expectations of another person. But rather than being completely self-absorbed, there is interaction with things and the world. So, there is lots of activity, fascination with anything new, and responsiveness to novelty, activity, movement, and, in particular, repetition, until a skill is fully acquired. This repetition is where the term 'practising' comes from. The child is practising by repetition, until a skill becomes part of their repertoire. Then a new skill is practised, and so on. People with severe and profound disabilities will have a limited range of skills that they can practise, but close observation will show that there are some. These may be as simple as blinking, pushing out the tongue, moving one hand or finger, and similar minimal activities – but these are activities that have meaning. I remember many years ago working with a profoundly disabled young child and discovering that he had voluntary control of the lower part of one arm. This was not immediately obvious until we gave him a skill to practise and he could pull a toy towards him if the string was attached to his arm. Clearly, a detail of this nature can be significant to the way that the child interacts with the world. Prior to this there was no awareness that he had voluntary control of anything.

As soon as we accept that the person, adult or child, is stuck at the practising stage, the intervention needs to be concentrating on facilitating development to the next stage. This is not to try to traverse the practising stage too quickly, but to remember that the aim is always to facilitate further development. Games feature in the practising stage, construction activities, and anything that raises awareness of surroundings. Reliable support and attention are essential. No one would leave a one-year-old child without adult support, and someone, of whatever age, who is stuck at the practising stage has the same need to know who the responsible adult is at any moment in time. So, a named member of staff must always be allocated. This does not mean they have to be in close contact at all time, but they must be available, and the client must know where their key person is. Activities such as going for a walk, to note the fact that you are walking, going up and down curbs, noticing traffic or plants or flowers, is a way of helping the individual to engage with the activity, the world and the person they are with. This comes very naturally with a one-year-old child, where you are increasing their interest in the world and what is going on around them. It comes less naturally when working with an older child or adult, but it is an essential part of an intervention. It is important as well to be patient as the person seeks to master the activity through their practising behaviour. So rather than take away an activity that is not working, it is better to persevere and help the individual to become competent. For example, if the task is building blocks and they keep falling down because of the difficulty with balancing them, it would be possible to do a hand-over-hand intervention to help the person to learn how to do it, to be successful, and to be successful in a joint activity. The practising stage, sadly, can sometimes be described as attention seeking, as the child or adult in the practising stage does need a lot of attention in order to keep trying to acquire the skills they are practising. If they do not get the attention that they need during this stage the range of activities reduces and, in worst-case scenarios, they will regress to the differentiation stage, engage in self-stimulating behaviour and stop trying.

The indications, and perhaps the main indication, of a movement from practising to early rapprochement is the shift to more two-way interaction. So, if you pass the ball to the child or adult, and they pass it back, they are engaging in two-way interaction. At the practising stage they would keep it and perhaps put their hand out for another one, but would not have any interest in passing it backwards and forwards. Peekaboo games and similar games can be used to encourage the move to the early rapprochement stage.

Early rapprochement

The early rapprochement stage is equivalent to the 15- to 24-month period of neurotypical development. Clearly it varies from child to child, but this is a rough guide. It is a time of rapid development and the beginnings of serious engagement with other people, hence leading to social development. People who are stuck in the early rapprochement stage still need lots of security over who is available for them, but they are much more challenging, and testing boundaries a lot of the time. Their behaviour almost always has a huge communication aspect to it. So, the behaviour is designed to make contact, to test out who is available and reliable, and, overall, to establish rapprochement i.e. two-way interaction. Again, these behaviours can be described as attention seeking, but as they have come to value interaction with others; it is better described as attention needing. If this stage is going well, then the individual is relaxed and engaged a lot of the time in positive two-way interaction. If it is not going well, then the person will be distressed and engaged in lots of what looks like attention seeking behaviour, demanding behaviour, and may be considered not very nice to be with. Of all the assessments of people with challenging behaviour that I have seen over many years of clinical practice, the majority of them are stuck in the early rapprochement stage. A significant number, also, are stuck between practising and early rapprochement. If we consider this from the point of view of ordinary development, this is the stage at which the child becomes more demanding and less easy to pacify. They also sleep less, which puts an additional pressure on their caregivers.

So, a programme of work with somebody stuck at the early rapprochement stage would involve structure, certainty, with a wide range of activities and social opportunities, and lots of social praise. They work well with a planned timetable. I've always found it very helpful to draw up a daily timetable of half-hour slots from 7am to 10pm, with one of the slots in the evening allocated to making the plan for the following day. It is important that there is an activity in each half-hour slot, even though the activity may only take a few minutes. This is to ensure that nothing is overtaxing, and that there is always something to look forward to. Once the pattern of saying what is going to happen and then making sure it does happen has become established, it becomes possible to put in place activities that are of benefit to learning. So, for example, putting in the morning routine of getting up, getting dressed, cleaning teeth, eating breakfast, and so on, will fill the first four or five slots. The next few can contain educational or practical activities, with one for a mid-morning drink, and then going on to the lunchtime break. Continuing in this way puts structure and order into the day, removes uncertainty and anxiety about what comes next, and provides opportunities for success. So, finding eating your breakfast is a success provides the individual with positive regard, and reduces anxiety in the interaction. Preparing breakfast together is a rapprochement behaviour and further develops the positive relationship. Having the written plan removes the anxiety of the question 'what shall we do now?' because it has already been decided. This may sound a very simple thing to do but it is significantly effective. We can compare this to the structure and planned day that would be provided in a nursery. It is emotional security that is the factor that makes it work. There may be issues about an individual preferring some staff to others, which can be a difficulty in supported living or education establishments. If everyone can be geared to responding to the written material, it can reduce that difficulty somewhat. Ideally, all staff working with an individual stuck at this early emotional developmental stage will have had training in understanding the model. If they have not, they may be tempted to start trying to introduce rewards and punishment at the wrong stage. There is an argument that punishment is never right, but withdrawal of favour is punishment and needs to be given serious consideration when putting together any plan for someone who is emotionally developmentally delayed. There is no room for withdrawal of attention or affection as part of the planned support, if structured emotional support is what the formulation indicates is needed. It can be quite hard to keep being positive with someone who is so traumatised that they cannot give anything back, which is why staff support is an important factor in the overall provision.

Late rapprochement

The indication that someone is moving into late rapprochement comes when they begin to start bargaining. The skills of negotiation, of coping with 'if – then' come with more maturity. It indicates that the individual being supported can now recognise that the other person may have wishes and needs that can be taken into consideration. This is a very demanding stage and, if described pejoratively, would be described as manipulative. If we think about the two- to three-year-old child, or perhaps up to four, we can recognise how much effort they put into getting their own way. This is a natural developmental stage as they begin to take responsibility, within their capability, for getting their own needs met. And it can become a battle of wills. If we reflect on how we would support a young child to prepare them for going to school, we would put significant effort into helping them to see that they cannot have their own way all the time, but they can negotiate for what they want. They can also begin to think about what others might want, and why. So, the child who does not want to get into the car because it is hot or boring, but cannot see that getting into the car is required in order to get to where they want to be, has to be reasoned with. It is only in this stage of late rapprochement that reasoning starts to become part of the process. There is no point in trying to reason with anybody at the early stages. And it can be joyful helping someone to get to the reasoning stage, and to pass through it to a point where they can make their own decisions and be confident that they are good decisions. It can be quite useful to use 'stop, think, decide' as a technique in this stage. In a situation where the arousal level is rising, there can be an increase in tension in the other people present. If someone, a member of staff, with confidence says, 'Stop a minute, let's think about this and decide what you are going to do', there will be a reduction in tension, and an increase in positive interaction and planning. Individuals with more ability, for example, with mild IDs, can learn to do it themselves, speaking to themselves with self-talk, and learn to regulate their emotions and behaviour. But again, it is only in this late rapprochement stage or after individuation that they can use the skill, so there is no point in using it, or trying to use it, with people who are more emotionally delayed.

The late rapprochement stage is quite long and quite hard, but it is very rewarding. I was taught many years ago that people behaved the way they did because of their disability. And it can be argued that their emotional disability accounts for their behaviour. Whereas the cognitive disability, which may be caused by brain damage, may not be able to be changed, the emotional disability can be. It was discovering this that fundamentally changed my way of working with people with disabilities. And the results have been significant and, at times, dramatic. If we take into consideration the cause of the emotional developmental delay, we come to a recognition of the impact of trauma. It follows that people who are stuck at the late rapprochement stage, and have developed the ability to work with someone else in two-way interaction, may benefit from individual psychological therapy. This is the fourth component of the model for treating people with emotional developmental delay and not everyone needs it. It would be good to do some formal research at some point and see if there is a relationship between the type of trauma and the type of response. It may be that people who are traumatised within the family after growing up with the pain of difference may be different from people who have been traumatised by third-party assault. However, my clinical practice, so far, would indicate that whatever the cause, treatment that takes account of the stage of emotional development is essential. Some people need individual therapy as well, and some do not, but if their basic needs for emotional support are not met, individual therapy will have limited impact.

Mahler describes something that she calls the rapprochement crisis. This is the point at which the individual becomes individuated, and it can be with a major tantrum that looks like a crisis or can be a shrug of the shoulders and acceptance. If we think about the three-and-a-half-year-old in neuro-typical development, we can think about the day that the child realises that their mother is not there, but they are OK with that. If we reflect on the nursery situation, where we can see some children constantly looking for who is there for them – some children will be happily playing and taking no notice of who is there – we can see the ones who are individuated and clear about their boundaries with the world (Winnicott's, 1971, me/not me boundary), then the difference is very clear.

Lots of people with intellectual disabilities do emotionally individuate, although they may still have to be dependent on others because of their limited cognitive, social or physical ability. They are quite different in their support needs from people who have not individuated. I sometimes think that that is why staff are confused when people of similar ability cognitively clearly do not have the ability to maintain relationships and live a relatively peaceful life.

Summary

In considering interventions with the model of emotional development, we can see that matching correctly is essential. The Frankish assessment of the impact of trauma (FA IT) has been developed specifically to measure and allocate the right stage. It is a simple and quick process, although there is a little bit of time needed to acquire confidence to make the judgements on what is observed. The method itself was thoroughly researched and found to be both reliable and valid. It takes 40 minutes, observing for 20 seconds, and writing for 40 seconds. Then the observations are rated one to four. The stage with the highest number of checks is the allocated stage. It is not uncommon to find that practising and early rapprochement are close in numbers. This seems to link with the number of people who are traumatised at the 12- to 18-month stage. It is impossible to know unless a study of nursery-age children is commissioned, but it is likely to link with the stage that parents begin to expect more from their child; with the arrival of a sibling; and the beginning of separation for nursery. If the assessment indicates a 'cusp' then the intervention needs to be planned for the practising stage and there will be fairly rapid transition to the next stage.

It is worth noting that the behaviour can look almost the same for all four stages. So, for example, if we consider a behaviour such as an individual hitting their own head. If it is recorded as hitting own head it could be a differentiation behaviour and self-referenced, so it is best to record it as, 'Hitting own head, not looking at anyone'. If it is recorded as, 'Hitting own head rhythmically', it is practising. If recorded as, 'Hitting own head, looking at staff', it is early-rapprochement and designed to communicate distress to another person. If recorded as, 'Hitting own head viciously', then it is late rapprochement and has the message, 'You had better do something', so it is calling for help. In my experience, people have learned quite quickly to make these distinctions.

This approach is not incompatible with others. It is possible to put the interventions into a positive behaviour support (PBS) format (chapter 8). What matters is the repeat assessment to ensure that the programme of support changes with the development and that it is understood. If the wrong approach is used at the wrong time, there will be serious consequences for the individual as the mismatch may activate past trauma of being unseen, unheard and uncared for. This can then lead to a breakdown in behaviour, displays of anger, and then a move to higher security. Or sometimes, to going back into a withdrawn state.

There are also similarities with intensive interaction (Chapter 9). The principle is the same, to make real human contact with another person who has given up on expecting positive human contact. It is perhaps less intensive, but it is meant to cover the whole 24 hours a day. Making sure that distressed people know who is there for them all the time, including who will be there when they wake up, is more than many have had for many years. It is possible to see, from this understanding, why some people like to be in segregation. They know where they stand, they know staff will always be there and they feel safe. If this emotional security is provided in good time, the escalation to segregation can be avoided. Understanding the very early emotional stage helps with the recognition of the primitive unconscious drives that maintain distressed behaviour for so many years, as we see in some individuals.

Similarly, there are clear links with attachment theory (Chapters 6 & 10). It is the quality of the attachments that facilitate recovery. Having a model that defines appropriate intervention that can be carried out by trained and supported support staff allows for more people to be helped than could be the case with intense one-to-one therapy. Providing the emotional secure base that Bowlby (1988) talks about, with the person-centered and specific emotional environment that Mahler writes about, in the model of trauma-informed care (TIC) that I have exercised my work, gives us a meaningful life opportunity for some very distressed and challenging people with IDs.

References

Bowlby J (1988) *A Secure Base*. London: Routledge.

Frankish P (2016) *Disability Psychotherapy*. London: Karnac.

Frankish P (2019) *Frankish Assessment of the Impact of Trauma*. London: Pavilion.

Frankish P (2019) *Trauma Informed Care: a guide for staff.* London: Pavilion.

Frankish P (2019) *Nought to Three – Becoming Me*. London: Pavilion.

Frankish P (1992) A psychodynamic approach to emotional difficulties within a social framework. *Journal of Intellectual Disability Research* **36** 559-563.

Frankish, P (1989) Meeting the emotional needs of handicapped people: A psychodynamic approach. *Journal of Mental Deficiency Research* **33**, 407-414.

Mahler M, Pine F & Bergman A (1979) *The Psychological Birth of the Human Infant*. New York: Basic.

Winnicott DW (1965) *Maturational Processes and the Facilitating Environment*. London: Karnac.

Winnicott DW (1971) *Playing and Reality*. London: Tavistock.

Winnicott DW (1973) *The Child, The Family and the Outside World*. Middlesex: Penguin.

Chapter 13:
Insults and spears: the tribulations of forensic disability psychotherapy

Brett Kahr

'Haven't you got a more normal patient?'

Many decades ago, I had the privilege of studying for several years at the famous Portman Clinic in London, an institution which, since the early 1930s, has specialised in providing psychoanalytical treatment for patients who have perpetrated acts of criminality. As a fledgling forensic psychotherapist, I deeply appreciated the opportunity to learn from such a distinguished group of senior mental health practitioners and I valued this opportunity immensely.

During my second year, I embarked upon regular weekly clinical supervision with one of the most experienced members of staff, whom I shall call 'Dr Jones' – a woman trained in both psychiatry and psychoanalysis. I became rather excited, knowing that I would learn a great deal from this extremely sophisticated clinician.

One day, I undertook an assessment of a male forensic patient who had attacked several elderly women in the street. In view of his violent assaults on innocent bystanders, this man had no difficulty meeting the diagnostic criteria as a proper forensic client. But, moreover, this gentleman, whom I shall call 'Riccardo', also battled with long-standing physical and intellectual disabilities. Back in those days, we referred to such patients as 'mentally handicapped'. Riccardo suffered from a congenital limp and from a degenerative ocular disease. which made walking rather difficult. Moreover, he struggled to speak clearly due to an early head injury, inflicted by a violent parent. Riccardo appeared extremely handicapped indeed and I had to listen very carefully in order to decipher his somewhat garbled language. With eager anticipation, I presented the case of Riccardo to my distinguished supervisor, hoping that I would become deeply enlightened, especially in view of Dr Jones's multi-decade experience of treating aggressive, forensic patients. But, to my surprise, this supervisor responded with a sense of alarm: 'Gosh, Brett, this chap is so mentally handicapped. He can barely free-associate as he is not at all verbally fluent. Haven't you got a more normal patient?'

The reaction of Dr Jones shocked me greatly. I knew that she had treated arsonists, rapists, paedophiles and murderers aplenty. But, as I soon came to discover, she had very little knowledge about, or experience of, those patients with an intellectual disability (ID). I discussed this matter with the course director, Dr Estela Welldon (subsequently Professor Welldon), who advised me to present a non-handicapped case instead. As an obliging young student, I did so, and Dr Jones proved most helpful. Alas, back in those days, few mental health practitioners, however sagacious, had an appetite to treat people diagnosed as disabled in any way.

At approximately the same time, I had the wonderful opportunity to work alongside Valerie Sinason, a blue-sky child psychotherapist at the Tavistock Clinic – only a stone's throw away from the Portman Clinic – and I joined both her Mental Handicap Team and her Mental Handicap Workshop. Sinason, along with other colleagues such as Neville Symington and, also, Jon Stokes, had pioneered the use of psychoanalytical psychotherapy as a treatment for the handicapped and disabled. But, alas, they aroused considerable suspicion from their Tavistock Clinic colleagues. Indeed, when I spoke to Dr Malcolm Pines (1996), who had worked alongside Neville Symington during the 1970s, I learned that many staff expressed tremendous suspicion about the use of verbal psychotherapy for those patients described at that time as 'subnormal', uncertain how one could truly deploy the Freudian 'talking cure' with patients who simply could not speak.
Fortunately, Valerie Sinason (1992; 2010) and other colleagues (e.g. Hollins, 1990a; 1990b; 1997; 2002; Corbett, 2014; Frankish, 2016; cf. Hollins & Sinason, 2000) persevered with the development of the discipline that we have since come to refer to as 'disability psychotherapy'.

In spite of the growth of this field, very few disability psychotherapists have worked extensively with forensic patients who also display handicaps of either a physical or intellectual nature. By contrast, although a considerable portion of mental health professionals have acquired an expertise in working with forensic cases, very few have developed a capacity for treating those who also suffer with disabilities.

Over the years, the field of disability psychotherapy has flourished, as has the discipline of forensic psychotherapy. But, only a very small handful of colleagues have worked on the complicated intersection between these two areas of speciality, which we have now come to refer to as *'forensic disability psychotherapy'* (Kahr, 2014; cf. Kahr, 2018; 2020).

Although I cannot do justice to the complex, but rewarding, arena of forensic disability psychotherapy in such a brief context, I will endeavour to provide a small flavour of how a mental health practitioner might engage a patient who meets the criteria for both intellectual disability and, also, criminality, by discussing the case of 'Tobiasz'.

Psychotherapy with a disabled genital exhibitionist: The handicapped film star

Long, long ago, an 18-year-old man named 'Tobiasz', recently cautioned by the police for genital exhibitionism, entered my consulting room in order to consider the possibility of undergoing psychotherapy. His father, 'Mr. X', accompanied Tobiasz for this very first appointment.

An extremely handsome young person with the classical looks of a film star, Tobiasz sported a highly exaggerated smile – quite often a characteristic defence against sadness and trauma (Sinason, 1986) – and he grinned at me broadly. After he responded to my invitation to sit down in the chair, his handicap, by no means visible from his striking physical appearance, soon became quite apparent.

'I … uh … I … uh … uhhhh … uhhhh … uuuhhh …'

Tobiasz fumbled and stumbled, unable to articulate a coherent sentence. I did not know to what extent his inability to speak with clarity stemmed from any baseline organic disability or, rather, from his anxiety about sitting across from a suited, bespectacled stranger in a potentially frightening context. Fortified by my prior teaching and supervision from Valerie Sinason (1986; 1992), I knew that an intensification of the patient's handicap could often mask a fear of communication. Hopeful that Tobiasz might begin to speak more fully and clearly, I smiled benignly and nodded patiently as this young person struggled to find some simple words.

The patient then opened his mouth and attempted to talk once again.

'I … uh … uh … I … ahhh … uhhh … I …'

At this point, I made a comment that it might be quite frightening for Tobiasz to have come to meet me, especially after having already undergone an interview with a policeman, at the police station, some weeks previously. I underscored that Tobiasz might be worried that I, too, could become a policeman who might send him to prison.

Apparently, the young man seemed relieved that I already knew something about his cautionary interview with the authorities, whereupon he replied in simple but, also, clear tones.

'Yes. The puuuh … leees. Puuuh … leees.'

He struggled to vocalise the word 'police', but, in spite of his handicapped rendition, I could certainly understand these sounds.

Mr X, recognising his son's long-standing difficulty at speaking in words, began, quite spontaneously and helpfully, to provide some further background information.

'As you can see, my son is a very handsome fellow. All the girls want to marry him because he is so handsome. His mother and I have always thought that he should become a film star.'

At this point, Tobiasz began to smile and to giggle. and his face lit up with delight.

'Film star,' he chirped, in completely audible tones. He had absolutely no difficulty articulating the phrase 'film star', and I sensed that he must have uttered these words many times previously.

Mr X then explained that, from the age of two years or thereabouts, Tobiasz had begun to display some sort of developmental delay of an indistinct nature. The doctors in their home country in Eastern Europe could not agree upon a diagnosis. One physician thought that he might be autistic, others suspected some sort of intellectual disability. No one knew. But, clearly, Tobiasz demonstrated certain signs of difficulty with both speech and concentration.

At this point, I thanked Mr X for having introduced his son to me and for having provided me with such useful biographical background. I then turned to Tobiasz and asked whether he would be happy to speak to me privately so that the two of us could begin to discuss his situation in more detail.

With a huge grin on his face, he pointed his finger at his father and muttered: 'You go away.' Mr X sniggered affectionately, rose from his seat, shook my hand, and explained that he would be waiting for Tobiasz in his car, parked just outside of my office building.

Once Mr X had left the consulting room, Tobiasz looked at me with a wide-eyed expression which, I imagined, conveyed not only his anxiety about having to participate in a psychotherapy consultation but, also, perhaps, his relief that he could now enjoy some independence from his father.

Within seconds of Mr X's departure, Tobiasz pounded his chest and boasted: 'Film star. I be film star.'

I looked at this strikingly handsome chap – a cross between Paul Newman and Robert Redford – and I smiled softly as Tobiasz attempted to enhance his fragile ego structure by fantasising about himself as a movie icon.

With Mr X now safely out of earshot, I felt authorised to speak to Tobiasz in a more psychologically intimate manner and I risked a first interpretation.

'Your father has told us that both he and your mother are very proud of what a handsome young man you have always been and that you could be a film star. And you have just told me that *you* want to be a film star. But I think that a part of you must wonder whether this dream will ever come true. And, in recent months, you have been showing off your penis to several young women. Perhaps you worry that, unless you display your body in that more striking way, no one will look at you or notice you. A young man exposing his private parts in public will attract a great deal of attention, just as film stars do.'

At this point, Tobiasz's great big smile disappeared and he began to look more forlorn.

'I … very handsome.'

I replied that as his parents, and many others besides, had often commented on his pleasant physical appearance, Tobiasz certainly had a lot of confirmatory evidence about his good looks. But I wondered whether a part of him did not always feel quite so good looking.

'I … ugly too,' he whispered. To which I replied: 'Well, I would imagine that even though you look very handsome on the outside and you receive a lot of lovely compliments, I suspect that, on the inside, you do, perhaps, feel ugly at times, and that you may become very upset when you think you might be different from other boys.'

He wasted no time in explaining: 'Other boys … girlfriends. I … no.'

I attempted to flesh out his cryptic statement: 'You are letting me know how sad it is that other boys have pretty girlfriends but that you do not have a girlfriend. And that is very disappointing for you … even *angry*-making … especially when you have been told every day that you are so handsome.'

He responded mournfully: 'No girlfriend … no girlfriend.'

I wondered aloud whether Tobiasz might also feel rather lonely, in spite of the fact that his parents have always doted upon him.

My comment seemed to strike a chord, and I derived some hope knowing that, in a more private conversation, Tobiasz could not only understand my speech, but, moreover, that his speech had become increasingly clear. Having begun the consultation uttering little more than occasional para-minimal encouragers (sounds such as 'uhhh' and 'ahhh'), he could now utilise longer words such as 'girlfriend' and 'handsome', which he could articulate with evident clarity.

I underscored that, although Tobiasz and I had only just met for the first time, and although I did not know a great deal about him as yet, I did have a sense that, in spite of being very handsome, and in spite of having very attentive and generous parents who love him greatly, he might be very sad and very angry at times, that he may be different from the other boys. By wishing to be a film star, he might hope that everything will turn out magically well. And by having displayed his private parts in public he had found a way to be looked at, although this had placed him in a potentially very dangerous and destructive situation.

At this point, Tobiasz stopped grinning and he stared at me with a very sad expression. To my surprise, he intoned: 'I … uhhh … I … uhhh … not good what I did. Not good.'

As our first meeting began to draw to a close, I explained that, as he knew, the family doctor had recommended that it might be useful for Tobiasz to talk to me about his situation. I underscored that although he and I had not yet discussed his genital displays in full, he might be willing to tell me more about what had happened and about his feelings, and that he and I might convene in private, on a weekly basis, to think about his life and to see whether such conversations could be helpful.

'Helpful,' murmured Tobiasz. 'Helpful.'

We arranged to meet the following week at the very same time, and I asked this young man whether he felt able to communicate this information to his father or whether he might wish for me to telephone his father to confirm the next appointment time. Tobiasz seemed keen to keep Mr X out of the consulting room, and I had a sense that he wished to communicate only with me. He thus replied: 'I tell him. Next week. Same time.'

Unzipping the trousers

One week later, Tobiasz arrived at the appropriate hour and we embarked upon our second session. Tobiasz remained silent and, after a short interval, I asked him how he had experienced our first meeting during the previous week, and what thoughts, if any, had stayed in his mind.

'You nice man. Nice man.'

I replied that if he considered me to be a 'nice man', he might feel a bit more comfortable to talk to me about his life and his world in greater detail … especially about some of the more difficult experiences and feelings.

'Like my penis.'

Previously, Tobiasz had not articulated the word 'penis'. Clearly, he possessed a more considerable capacity for verbal communication than he had revealed during the opening moments of our first consultation.

I then invited him to tell me about the times when he had displayed his penis. Without hesitation, he explained that, one day, some three months previously, he found himself seated in the back row of the upper deck of a bus, and, while looking at a very pretty girl across the aisle, he became 'hard'. He told me, in a very unhandicapped manner, that he wanted the girl to touch his penis, and so he unzipped his trousers and exposed himself, thinking that she would find his genitals attractive. The girl – some 17 or 18 years of age – rose instantly from her seat and disappeared from view, with a look of horror on her face. Tobiasz explained that he felt very saddened by this rejection and could not understand why she would not play with his penis.

'So pretty,' he whimpered.

I commented that, although he had difficulty comprehending why the beautiful girl did not touch his private parts, as he had wished, perhaps he also struggled to appreciate that the young woman might have a mind of her own, and that, however handsome Tobiasz might be, he had probably scared this person by having exposed himself so abruptly.

He stuttered: 'Me not dane … dane … dane …'

'Dangerous?' I intoned.

'Me not dangerous,' Tobiasz underscored.

I explained that while he did not consider himself to be dangerous at all, it might be challenging to imagine that he may have had quite a frightening impact upon someone else.

He then revealed that, over the course of several weeks, he had 'unzipped' himself on four or five further occasions, always in the back row of the bus, and always in the presence of a pretty girl.

Although most of the young women to whom he exposed himself had walked away briskly in an act of self-protection, one of them ran to the driver, who stopped the bus and telephoned the police. Eventually, two officers escorted Tobiasz off the bus and then interrogated him.

He told me that he did not realise that the police would be so angry at him. Apparently, one of the policemen who removed Tobiasz from the bus pushed him rather aggressively, and this frightened him considerably. The young man could not understand why the officer had to be so 'mean'.

As I listened to Tobiasz, I became increasingly impressed that, in spite of his intellectual disability and his tendency to struggle verbally, he did manage to express himself with coherence and he could, albeit with some difficulty, narrate moments from his life history. This made me quite hopeful that we might eventually be able to learn something about his deeper motivations for these acts of genital exhibitionism.

Throughout this conversation, I became curious as to *when*, precisely, Tobiasz started to unzip his trousers. Had he done so for many years or had these illegal activities begun only quite recently? Tobiasz responded to my query in a very straightforward manner and he told me that he had never taken his penis out of his trousers until just a few months earlier, not long after his 18th birthday. I attempted to discover why he had begun to exhibit himself at this point, rather than one or two or three years previously. Having worked with other male genital exhibitionists in my practice, I knew that the act of exposure often emerged in response to specific traumata, and I wished to discover whether some particular event or fantasy had triggered Tobiasz's actions, hoping that our future sessions would offer further clarity.

I thanked this young man for having begun to speak to me about a very important and very scary set of experiences, which had resulted in a caution by the local police. I then underscored that, as our sessions progressed over the coming weeks, we would have an opportunity to think in more detail about these and many other biographical experiences so that we could acquire a better understanding of the workings of his mind.

As the months unfolded, Tobiasz and I continued our regular psychotherapeutic work. Over time, I learned a great deal more about Tobiasz's early childhood. He began to reminisce, free-associatively, about his sixth birthday party, for which his mother baked a delicious chocolate cake with vanilla icing and his father took him riding on a pony. He recalled how, during his eighth year, he began to listen to pop music on the radio and he particularly enjoyed the songs of The Beatles, especially the classic *Yellow Submarine*, which he then began to hum for me. He talked of his grandmother who doted upon him, and of his many aunts and uncles and cousins, all of whom treated him 'nice'. Unlike my other patients who have disabilities, many of whom suffered horrific traumata at the hands of parents or institutional staff members, Tobiasz seemed to have had an idyllic childhood. And yet, he had displayed his private parts in public, causing great distress to several young females, and he did evoke the serious concern of the police. What on earth propelled a boy from such a seemingly loving and sturdy family to behave in such a manner?

Exposing the trauma

After several months of work, Tobiasz had painted an increasingly detailed and verbally rich portrait of his early childhood. But, thus far, we had devoted very little time to his schooling. I learned that, for the first 10 years of his life, Tobiasz did not attend either a nursery or a primary school in his country of origin; instead, his wealthy parents paid for a tutor to educate him in the family residence, as the local physicians explained that 'retarded' children should be home-schooled. Tobiasz recalled a succession of very warm-hearted private tutors. Naturally, I had to entertain the possibility that one of these teachers might have harmed him in some way, but Tobiasz described each tutor in turn as a friendly and kindly person who taught him about letters and numbers and, also, about history.

During one of our sessions, I expressed a curiosity to this young patient as to whether he felt disappointed that he had not attended a traditional school like all the other boys and girls in his hometown. To my surprise, he told me that he did, in fact, become a 'boarder' at the age of 10, although he quickly clarified that he had done so, 'only for a bit … only for a bit'.

Over the course of several psychotherapy sessions, Tobiasz shared some fairly anodyne memories of his time at boarding school, recalling, for instance, that he had a nice set of pencils and pens and, also, some lovely crayons. But he never mentioned the other boys at this single-sex school, nor did he speak about any sadness at having had to leave his family.

Eventually, after months of regular, sustained psychotherapeutic work, Tobiasz entrusted me with a vital memory and shared a very 'big secret' that he had never revealed to anyone else before. I remained silent with a look of concern on my face, and, with a gentle nod of the head, I encouraged him to begin speaking, whereupon I learned that, not long after his arrival at the boarding school, the other 10-year-old boys began to tease him for being a 'retard' and for speaking in a slow and indistinct manner.

One night, after the teacher had turned off the lights in the large dormitory, the other boys – about six or seven of them – attacked Tobiasz. In an effort to shame him, they pinned him to the floor so that he could not move, and then they stuffed a sock in his mouth so that he could not scream, ultimately stripping him of all of his clothing. The tormentors proceeded to make fun of Tobiasz for having a 'little penis', and one of the more outspoken schoolmates humiliated him further by declaiming: 'Look, even his dick is retarded.' Most shocking of all, this gang decided that they would 'torture' Tobiasz by 'ripping off' his penis from his body, whereupon several of these abusive lads began to pull on his genitals, tugging quite viciously, for several minutes, so much so that Tobiasz actually thought that they would detach his penis completely.

This dreadful assault became an almost nightly ritual until, one day, Tobiasz received permission to telephone his parents and demanded that he be removed from the school. Sensing their son's unhappiness, the parents responded to his request and they returned him to the family home. But Tobiasz, full of shame at this castrating attack on his body and on his sense of self, had kept these episodes a complete secret, and neither his teachers nor his parents ever discovered what had happened to him.

Tobiasz became teary-eyed as he struggled to relate the details of this traumatic episode to me. To his credit, he did so in clear words, with much detail. At times, the tears simply streamed down his cheeks. Strikingly, he never reached for a tissue, readily available on a nearby shelf, and I commented that perhaps he had waited eight years for these tears to emerge and that by crying and by having shared this experience with me he might begin to feel some relief.

Although it would be far too simplistic to conceptualise psychoanalytical work as the simple revelation of a trauma, leading to an immediate recovery, Tobiasz's narration of the attack on his penis as a 10-year-old boy certainly produced a tremendous sense of catharsis. Subsequently, he spoke with even greater verbal fluidity, as though he had begun, at last, to find his voice.

In subsequent sessions, he and I reflected at great length about the impact of these episodes. We discussed his sense of shame at feeling 'like a girl', unable to fight back 'like a boy'. We explored his fear that the other boys hated him for being a 'retard' and, also, for having a rich and famous father. He also dared to suggest that, because he looked far more handsome than the other boys, they might have resented his appearance. Without having mentioned the word 'envy', Tobiasz certainly theorised with the clinical intelligence of a seasoned mental health practitioner.

Eventually, after Tobiasz spoke at greater length about these traumata, we then began to consider the potential impact of such an emotionally shocking and physically painful experience – the near loss of his penis – upon his subsequent acts of genital exhibitionism eight years later. Once we had established a connection between his boarding school abuse and his eventual exhibitionism, Tobiasz could begin to appreciate that he might have needed to display his penis in front of those 'pretty girls' who, he believed, would admire his genitals, in the hope of repairing the pain of the exposure of his private parts in front of those 'ugly boys'.

As we began to understand more and more about the deeply hurtful and profoundly shaming experiences that Tobiasz had endured as a boarder at school, he became increasingly able to discuss private matters in a more straightforward way. Gradually, we devoted greater consideration to an exploration of why his genital exhibitionism had emerged in his 18th year, rather than at some other time.

Although there may be many factors that contributed to this young man's exhibitionist activities at that particular moment, we did come to discover that, shortly before the first public exposure of his genitals, Tobiasz had experienced an emotionally castrating attack from a stranger. With tears in his eyes and rage in his voice, Tobiasz told me that, one day, while out for a stroll, a boy, no more than 14 or 15 years old, passed him on the pavement. Sensing that Tobiasz might have a learning difficulty of some sort, this young person began insulting him: 'You're a fucking faggot. You're a fucking retard.' Tobiasz did not retaliate; he simply continued on his walk. But he felt absolutely wretched. And only three or four days later, quite eviscerated and demasculinised, he displayed his penis on a bus for the very first time. Tobiasz enjoyed making connections of this sort and, gradually, he began to develop an infinitely richer understanding of his behaviours and his emotions.

After 14 months of sustained psychotherapy, I received a telephone call from the father, Mr X, informing me that a high-ranking official in his country of origin had invited him to return home to assume a new appointment and that, in consequence, he and his family would have to move back to Eastern Europe in two months' time. I must confess that this sudden announcement saddened me, as I had developed a great fondness for Tobiasz, quite impressed by his capacity for emotional growth. We had reached a point where he had become much more verbally fluent, much more insightful, and much more empathic, even expressing sadness that some of the girls might have found his penis scary. Fortunately, we had eight more sessions in which to prepare for an ending and to say goodbye.

In our final meeting, Tobiasz told me, quite touchingly, that he would miss me. I replied that I had appreciated the serious way in which he had committed himself to the psychotherapeutic process, that I would think about him afterwards, and that I hoped he would be well. Tobiasz parted with a warm handshake and with a look of deep kindness in his eyes.

Approximately six months after our psychotherapy ended, Tobiasz sent me a handwritten note, posted from his country of origin, in which he expressed his sincere thanks to me for our work together over the past year. To my relief and delight, he reassured me that, nowadays, while riding the bus, he behaves like 'a very nice man'. To the best of my knowledge, Tobiasz engaged in no further acts of public genital exhibitionism in the years that followed.

Transforming spears into insults

Forensic disability psychotherapy, a relatively new discipline within mental health, endeavours to provide compassionate, humane psychological treatment for those individuals who not only struggle with disabilities but who also engage in acts of criminality. Although every human being has the potential to commit an illegal act, some of our patients who have disabilities may, at times, be at risk of doing so, owing to their struggle with the sheer act of verbalisation. Many of these men and women must bear tremendous anger, often the result of trauma – and yet, owing to their lack of linguistic fluency, some will become more likely to enact these experiences through the perpetration of forensic activities.

In view of this, the practice of psychotherapy offers offenders with disabilities the possibility of long-term attachment repairs through ongoing treatment, and, also, provides an opportunity to verbalise hidden and repressed secrets and aggressions, helping to turn those unbearable affects into words, rather than actions.

In 1969, Dr Donald Winnicott, the noted English psychoanalyst, received a letter from a colleague who worked with mentally ill children, requesting advice on how to handle boys and girls who might curse (Balbernie, 1969; cf. Kahr, 1998). With sagacity, Winnicott (1969) replied, suggesting that the verbalisation of foul language might be a godsend: 'How much nicer is hate than murder and how silly we are if we mind when children scream out "fuck" and other obscenities.'

But no one encapsulated the vital role of talking more succinctly than the young neurologist, Dr Sigmund Freud (1893), who, quite early in his career, underscored that, 'as an English writer has wittily remarked, the man who first flung a word of abuse at his enemy instead of a spear was the founder of civilization'. Thus, if we can help our physically violent, spear-throwing forensic patients, whether disabled or not, to transform their actions into angry words or insults, we have the potentiality to make a small contribution towards helping the world enjoy greater peace and tranquillity.

Acknowledgements

I wish to express my warm thanks to Nigel Beail, Patricia Frankish, and Allan Skelly for their kind invitation to contribute a chapter to this edited volume. I published a more extended version of the case of 'Tobiasz' in an essay entitled, Penile Trauma and Genital Exhibitionism: From Castration Anxiety to Verbal Potency, which appeared in *The International Journal of Forensic Psychotherapy* (Kahr, 2019). I wish to extend my warmest thanks to the Joint Editors-in-Chief, Ms Jessica Collier and Carine Minne, and, also, to Mrs Kate Pearce, the Publisher of Phoenix Publishing House, for their kind permission to reproduce this clinical material (albeit in revised form) for this collection of essays.

References

Balbernie, R (1969) Letter to Donald W Winnicott. 17 March. Box 7, File 10, Donald W. Winnicott Papers in the Archives of Psychiatry, The Oskar Diethelm Library, DeWitt Wallace Institute of Psychiatry, Weill Cornell Medical College, New York.

Corbett, A. (2014) *Disabling Perversions: Forensic Psychotherapy with People with Intellectual Disabilities*. London: Karnac Books.

Frankish P (2016) *Disability Psychotherapy: An Innovative Approach to Trauma-Informed Care*. London: Karnac Books.

Freud S (1893) On the Psychical Mechanism of Hysterical Phenomena. In: S Freud (1962) *The Standard Edition of the Complete Psychological Works of Sigmund Freud: Volume III*. (1893-1899). *Early Psycho-Analytic Publications*. J Strachey, A Freud, A Strachey & A Tyson (Eds and Transls) (pp27–39). London: Hogarth Press and the Institute of Psycho-Analysis.

Hollins S (1990a). Group analytic therapy with people with mental handicap. In: A Došen, A van Gennep & GJ Zwanikken (Eds) *Treatment of Mental Illness and Behavioral Disorder in the Mentally Retarded: Proceedings of the International Congress. May 3 – 4, 1990. Amsterdam, The Netherland*s (pp81-89). Leiden: Logon Publications.

Hollins S.(1990b) Grief Therapy for People with Mental Handicap. In: A Došen, A van Gennep & GJ Zwanikken (Eds) *Treatment of Mental Illness and Behavioral Disorder in the Mentally Retarded: Proceedings of the International Congress. May 3 – 4, 1990. Amsterdam, The Netherlands* (pp81-89). Leiden: Logon Publications.

Hollins S (1997) Counselling and Psychotherapy. In: O Russell (Ed) *Seminars in the Psychiatry of Learning Disabilities* (pp245-258). London: Gaskell/Royal College of Psychiatrists.

Hollins S (2002) What is the future of the psychiatry of learning disability? *Psychiatric Bulletin: The Journal of Psychiatric Practice* 26 283–284.

Hollins S & Sinason V (2000) Psychotherapy, learning disabilities and trauma: New perspectives. *British Journal of Psychiatry* **176** 32–36.

Kahr B (1998). An Unpublished Fragment by Donald Winnicott. *NewSquiggle* **2**, 7.

Kahr B (2014). Series editor's foreword: Towards forensic disability psychotherapy. In: A Corbett *Disabling Perversions: Forensic Psychotherapy with People with Intellectual Disabilities* (ppxiii–xxii). London: Karnac Books.

Kahr B (2018) Estela at La Scala. In: B Kahr (Ed) *New Horizons in Forensic Psychotherapy: Exploring the Work of Estela V Welldon* (pp1-14). London: Karnac Books.

Kahr B (2019) Penile trauma and genital exhibitionism: From Castration Anxiety to Verbal Potency. *International Journal of Forensic Psychotherapy* **1** 93-108.

Kahr B (2020) *Dangerous Lunatics: Trauma, Criminality, and Forensic Psychotherapy*. London: Confer/Confer Books.

Pines M (1996) Personal Communication to the Author. 14 December.

Sinason V (1986) Secondary handicap and its relationship to trauma. *Psychoanalytic Psychotherapy* **2** 131–154.

Sinason V (1992) *Mental Handicap and the Human Condition: New Approaches from the Tavistock*. London: Free Association Books.

Sinason V (2010) *Mental Handicap and the Human Condition: An Analytic Approach to Intellectual Disability* (revised edition). London: Free Association Books.

Winnicott DW (1969) Letter to Richard Balbernie. 18 March. Box 7, File 10, Donald W. Winnicott Papers in the Archives of Psychiatry, The Oskar Diethelm Library, DeWitt Wallace Institute of Psychiatry, Weill Cornell Medical College, New York.

Chapter 14: Trauma-informed cognitive behavioural therapy

Biza Stenfert Kroese

Introduction

Previous chapters have already mentioned the wealth of evidence that people with intellectual disabilities (IDs) are not only more likely to be exposed to adverse life events that affect their physical and psychological health (Emerson and Brigham, 2014) but also are more likely to experience multiple traumatic events (Beadle-Brown *et al.,* 2010). Although the impact of experiencing more negative events on our clients is not, as yet, clearly understood, the consensus is that people with ID are more likely to suffer from post-traumatic stress disorder (PTSD) than the rest of the population (e.g. Daveney *et al.,* 2019).

The trauma experienced may be as a direct consequence of having a disability, such as perpetrators being more likely to target vulnerable people (Byrne, 2018), or being separated from family at an early age and experiencing multiple residential placements. Also, people with ID are more likely to be exposed to a number of social factors that are determinants of (general but also mental) health: poverty, poor housing, unemployment, social exclusion and overt discrimination (Emerson and Hatton, 2007). Added to this, the distress that is caused by PTSD symptoms may be compounded by cognitive deficits and a lack of effective coping skills, as well as limited access to mental health services (Stenfert Kroese *et al.,* 2013). Yet another disadvantage for people with ID is that, even if they are fortunate enough to be offered a mental health service, their PTSD may go undetected by the professionals they encounter. When people have limited ability to express themselves (and so struggle to talk about their feelings and thoughts), it is difficult to find out what the underlying psychological experiences are that are causing their distress. And a lack of specialist training and, to date, the weak and tentative evidence-base for suitable and effective interventions (Byrne, 2020; Stenfert Kroese *et al.,* 2016; Truesdale *et al.,* 2019) further contribute to the challenges faced by mental health clinicians working with people with ID.

That relatively few people with ID are given access to mental health services is not only due to a lack of training on mental health issues (including the impact of trauma on mental health) received by staff working in specialist ID services, but also a lack of knowledge and experience of ID on the part of generic mental health professionals (Stenfert Kroese *et al.,* 2013). Although the majority of professional and support staff working in ID services come in regular contact with service users who have mental health problems, a minority receive training in this complex area (Rose, Kent and Rose, 2012) yet evidence indicates that even brief training can increase confidence, attitudes and working practices in staff (Costello, Bouras and Davies, 2007). It is particularly important that front-line workers are able to recognise the symptoms of mental illness, especially PTSD, and have the confidence to refer to specialist services when needed, as often service users themselves do not have the ability or opportunity to self-refer.

On a more positive note, and evidenced by this book, we have recently seen a definite surge in trauma-focused treatments that have been adapted to make them accessible for people with ID. In this chapter, I will describe some of the trauma-focused cognitive behavioural therapy (TF-CBT) approaches that have been developed and how these may be used to benefit people with trauma-induced mental health problems who also have an ID. I will also touch on some of the quantitative and qualitative methods that have been used to collect evidence of acceptability and effectiveness of these clinical approaches, and ways forward in research methodology. But first, I want to summarise what we know about the impact of traumatic events on our clients with ID, as this has important implications for the ways in which clinicians approach their work.

Impact of trauma

As a clinician, I have observed remarkable resilience in some clients but for many people with ID traumatic events are not easily dealt with and can lead to enduring PTSD or complex trauma (Brewin *et al.,* 2000). The high levels of exposure to trauma and subsequent long-term distress suffered by our clients clearly indicate that, as clinicians who work with people with ID, we should have trauma at the front of our minds and that we have a responsibility to become skilled in, and widely practice, trauma-informed interventions.

But do we know whether for adults with ID the psychological impact of experiencing trauma is similar or the same as for the general population? We have some initial evidence for a relationship between trauma and reduced psychological well-being in people with ID. A longitudinal study of 68 adults with ID found a relationship between adverse life events (ALES[1]) as measured by the Bangor Life Events Schedule for ID and psychological and behavioural problems at follow-up (Hulbert-Williams, Hastings, Owen *et al.,* 2014). Also, in a prospective study ALES were found to predict psychological trauma for 99 adults with mild and moderate ID assessed six months later, as measured by the Lancaster and Northgate Trauma Scales (Wigham, Taylor and Hatton, 2014).

A recent retrospective study (Morris *et al.,* 2020) on the impact of exposure to adverse childhood events (ACES) in 36 adolescents with developmental disabilities, who were detained in a secure specialist in-patient facility, found that almost all had experienced at least one ACE, more than half had experienced four or more, and a third had six or more ACES. The most common types of ACES reported were physical abuse, parental separation and emotional abuse. The majority of these young people had also experienced high levels of disruption during their lives, with an average of four placement breakdowns (and a staggering range of one to 13). ACES were significantly and positively correlated with the number of placement breakdowns as well as with the number of mental health diagnoses with which the young people had been labelled.

As part of a qualitative, explorative study of the impact of trauma, Mitchell, Clegg and Furniss interviewed six adults with mild ID from a clinical population about their experiences of trauma. They found that their participants had experienced long-term effects that were similar to those reported in the general population (e.g. Steil and Ehlers, 2000), including a permeating and distressing belief that their and/or others' lives were in danger. Participants also reported intrusive mental images related to the trauma and some talked about seeing such images when they were trying to get to sleep. Non-disabled traumatised adults also report that re-experiencing of a traumatic event usually takes the form of visual images and often just before or during sleep (Ehlers and Clark, 2000). Mitchell *et al*'s (2006) participants also stated that they often used avoidance strategies for fear of something bad happening again, very similar to case reports of people without ID. We know that avoidance can reduce anxiety and distress in the short-term but that it can have a severely limiting and isolating effect on a person's lifestyle, which can

---

1   Adverse life or childhood events (ALES and ACES) are used here as broad terms that refer to a wide range of circumstances or events that pose a serious threat to physical or psychological well-being. Trauma is defined here as experiencing a specific event or set of circumstances as extremely frightening, harmful, or threatening. These terms will be used interchangeably as they fit on continua of duration and range.

cause additional psychological as well as social problems for the person and those around them in the longer-term.

A study (Mason-Roberts *et al.,* 2018) of 33 adults with ID and a diagnosis of PTSD found that the participants who reported that they had experienced ALES as well as ACES suffered greater psychological distress, and displayed more challenging and self-injurious behaviours compared with those who reported exposure to ALES only. They concluded that more severe psychological problems in adulthood are associated with multiple traumas in childhood and adulthood, compared with trauma experienced in adulthood only.

Some authors (e.g. Byrne, 2018) have questioned whether the concept of PTSD and its symptoms can be applied to people with ID and, for this reason, Mason-Roberts *et al.*, (2018) have argued that there is a need to further research the phenomenology and standardisation of instruments that are suitable for our client group. The most recent ICD-11 includes a new condition, complex PTSD, which is associated with previous multiple traumas (Karatzias *et al.,* 2017). There is now an urgent need for research that can determine whether this new classification and method of assessment can be used for people with ID and, if not, whether modifications can make them thus.

In short, we do not yet have sufficient information about the exact impact of trauma on people with ID, although a number of studies have identified very similar psychological consequences for people with ID as those observed in the general population.

Trauma-specific treatments

The psychological problems of adults with ID who have experienced traumatic events and who subsequently experience PTSD have, until recently, been typically managed pharmacologically, although there is no clear evidence that such drug treatment actually works (Stenfert Kroese, Dewhurst and Holmes, 2001; Willner, 2015) or by working behaviourally with staff teams to modify their environment for which there is good evidence (British Psychological Society, 2018). But it is important to stress that neither of these types of intervention have been designed to understand and address in detail the underlying causes of PTSD, as talking therapies can do.

There is now a growing body of research that has focused on the feasibility and efficacy of trauma-specific talking therapies for people with ID. This type of treatment directly targets the psychological and inter-personal problems that result from ALES and ACES. The interventions that have been researched most methodically and which have been shown to have some efficacy are grounded in or are used in conjunction with a cognitive behavioural therapy (CBT) model. They are usually referred to as trauma-focused cognitive behavioural therapy (TF-CBT; Cohen, Mannarino and Murray, 2011) and eye movement desensitisation and reprocessing (EMDR; Shapiro, 1999).

CBT was developed by Aaron Beck (Beck, Rush, Shaw, and Emery, 1979) and is based on a combination of behavioural and cognitive principles. CBT focuses on the relationships between thoughts, emotions, and behaviours. Its core assumption is that improvements in psychological well-being can result from changes in cognitions – that is, how we think has an influence on how we feel and behave. Beck explained his CBT theory in terms of errors in information processing. People's distress is caused by their errors in interpreting the meaning of events, which can result in catastrophising or overgeneralising, and developing a bias for particular cues. Underlying these processing errors are 'schema', which are assumptions about oneself and the world. Schema are described as underlying cognitive structures that can create vulnerability to mental health problems, because they act as templates for the perception, encoding, storage, and retrieval of information. Negative schema can lie 'dormant' for some time until they are triggered by particular events that make people think along the lines of their underlying negative schema. In Beck's work on depression, the core schemata include 'a negative triad', with depressed people holding negative views about themselves, their current life, as well as their future.

Jeffrey Young (Young, 1999) elaborated on Beck's theory and developed schema-focused cognitive therapy. According to this theory, early maladaptive schema (EMS) about yourself and your relationships with others can develop during childhood and throughout your lifetime. They are made up of memories and cognitions and, when they are activated, intense emotions are felt. These schema-focused principles can be applied to explain and treat trauma-related psychological symptoms. The errors of information processing (or schema) that are most likely to follow childhood trauma are 1) *over-vigilance and inhibition* (expecting that things will go wrong at any moment and a focus on controlling and suppressing your emotions and spontaneous feelings so as to avoid things going wrong or making mistakes) and 2) *disconnection and rejection* (expecting that your needs for safety, stability, empathy and respect will not be met by important others), both of which can result in serious long-term problems in mental health and interpersonal functioning (Tezel, Kislac and Boysan, 2015).

Authors who have adopted and researched TF-CBT recommend that people with complex trauma respond best to phase-based treatment with an initial stabilisation phase to learn coping skills, then a trauma processing phase to understand personal trauma experiences, and a final integration phase to consolidate and generalise safety and trust (e.g. Ford *et al.,* 2005; Murray, Cohen, Ellis and Mannarino, 2008).

EMDR, developed by Shapiro (1999; 2001), aims to resolve symptoms that are caused by traumatic experiences and that remain unprocessed. EMDR involves asking the client to attend to the emotionally disturbing memories while simultaneously focusing on an external stimulus, typically in the form of guided bilateral eye movement or tapping. The underlying theory assumes an interaction of cognitions, emotions and bodily sensations linked with the memory of the traumatic experience. The core feature of the EMDR procedure is receiving bilateral stimulation while concentrating on the trauma memory. Concentrating on the images and negative cognitions that arise is meant to enable the client access to the emotional and somatic aspects of the memory. During the bilateral stimulation, the therapist asks the client to 'go with' whatever arises from their awareness. The client is asked repeatedly to report emotional, cognitive, somatic experiences, and images until they can report a subjective unit of disturbance (SUD) of zero and adaptive and positive beliefs are rated as 'strong' on a validity of cognition scale.

The underlying information processing theory is based on the assumption that the application of EMDR induces a physiological condition in which unprocessed memories of traumatic events become linked up with networks made up of adaptive information and skills (Shapiro, 2007). Various experimental studies support this theory by showing that eye movements during recall of aversive memories reduce their vividness and emotionality (Engelhart *et al.,* 2011). During recall, emotional memories become 'labile' and their reconsolidation is affected by experiences during recall (Baddeley, 1998). Recalling a traumatic memory is assumed to tax working memory capacity, which is limited. If another task (such as guided eye movements) is carried out during recall, less capacity will be available in working memory for recalling a distressing event. This results in the memory being experienced as less vivid and emotional, and so more easily tolerated.

Although both TF-CBT and EMDR are treatments for trauma that are based on convincing theoretical models backed up by experimental evidence, as well as robust outcome research for the general population, we now need to consider the evidence that exists for their application in ID services.

The evidence so far for TF-CBT and EMDR for people with ID

In Ehlers and Clark's (2000) CBT model, PTSD develops when people process trauma in a way that leads to a sense of serious, current threat. Sense of threat is influenced by excessively negative appraisals of the trauma itself and the consequences of the trauma. The nature of the trauma memory is also implicated in that, if a person has a poorly elaborated and contextualised memory, they are more likely to experience PTSD. McNally and Shin (1995) found that people with low intellectual ability process memories in terms of sensory impressions rather than processing the meaning and context of the event. They propose this as an explanation for the higher incidence of PTSD in people with ID.

CBT has been adapted for people with mild ID and has been shown to be effective in the treatment of mood disorders, anxiety disorders, and aggression (e.g. Taylor *et al.,* 2013; Willner and Hatton, 2006), with effect sizes comparable to those reported in the general population (Vereenooghe and Langdon, 2013; Willner and Lindsay, 2016). CBT has also been shown to be highly valued by service users and their carers (e.g. Pert *et al.,* 2013; Stenfert Kroese *et al.,* 2016). One user's view of CBT was: 'I talk about it more now and I feel a lot better, relaxed. I feel this great big weight come off my shoulders and I feel thingy, and that weight can stay away altogether and I feel a lot better' (Pert *et al.,* 2013). So we are now reasonably confident that CBT can be an effective and acceptable treatment for people with ID with a variety of psychological problems.

But although CBT approaches are the most researched of all therapies for people with ID and PTSD, and shown to be well tolerated and associated with improvement in mental health (Keesler, 2020), no controlled studies have yet been conducted on their efficacy. We do have some evidence (despite methodological criticisms) from case studies that EMDR is associated with improvements in mood, physical well-being, and increased skills in people with ID (Gilderthorp, 2015; Mevissen *et al.,* 2011a&b; 2012; 2017).

Unwin *et al.* (2019) investigated process issues for the implementation of EMDR. Semi-structured interviews were conducted with two adults with ID and three clinical psychologists who had participated in EMDR as well as a key supporter. The interviews were analysed thematically and five themes were identified: EMDR feels very different; EMDR is a technical process; the need to work with the present; talking is important; cautious optimism. They concluded that whilst a range of client- and therapist-related factors served as barriers to using EMDR (such as a preference for working with the present rather than with memories), they felt cautiously optimistic that EMDR may be useful for 'the right person at the right time'.

A recent review of published case reports in which CBT and/or EMDR techniques were used for treating PTSD symptoms (Byrne, 2020) also suggest promise. Byrne appraised the effectiveness of both CBT and EMDR for PTSD and associated symptoms in adults and children with ID. A systematic search identified 11 papers published between 2010 and March 2020, eight focused on EMDR and three on CBT. He judged the methodological quality of these papers to be weak, but concluded tentatively that EMDR and CBT are both acceptable and feasible treatment options for both adults and children with ID, although no firm conclusions can be drawn about effectiveness because of small sample sizes, a lack of standardised assessments, and a dearth of controlled designs. Byrne's review confirms that further research is needed to provide evidence for treatment effectiveness and the modifications needed to make these treatment approaches suitable for people with ID.

Some clinical experiences

I will devote this next section to describing some clinical experiences of applying TF-CBT[2] and attempts to assess whether these methods actually benefit our clients.

Some time ago, we (Stenfert Kroese and Thomas, 2006) described two case studies that used imagery rehearsal therapy (IRT) with two young women with ID who had been sexually, physically and emotionally abused, and who suffered from frequent PTSD nightmares and flashbacks of the abuse. IRT is based on CBT principles and the assumptions that:

1. nightmares can be caused by traumatic events and sometimes serve a beneficial purpose immediately following trauma by providing information and emotional processing

2. nightmares persisting for months no longer serve a useful purpose

3. repetitive nightmares are habits or learned behaviours and can be treated as such

---

2   For a detailed overview of suitable adaptations to make a wide variety of CBT techniques not specifically focused on trauma but accessible to people with ID, refer to Jahoda, Stenfert Kroese and Pert (2017) and Stenfert Kroese (2014).

4. working with waking imagery influences nightmares because things thought about during the day are related to things dreamed about at night

5. nightmares can be changed into positive, new imagery

6. rehearsing new imagery (a new dream) while awake reduces or eliminates nightmares.

The standard IRT protocol (Krakow *et al.,* 2001) is to ask clients to explore the possibility that although nightmares may be trauma-induced, they may also be habit-sustained. They then practice pleasant imagery exercises and learn to deal with unpleasant images that might emerge. During the next stage, they learn how to use IRT on a PTSD nightmare. They are asked to write down the disturbing dream, then to change the nightmare any way they wish and to write down the changed dream. Afterward, they rehearse the new dream for 10 to 15 minutes and are advised to repeat this exercise every day.

We have adapted this protocol to make it accessible and acceptable for our clients with ID. Instead of writing down the nightmare and the new dream, we work together with the client to draw the dream sequence and talk through the events. Drawings are included for two main reasons. First, the use of art in dream work appears to help people remember and work through childhood abuse experiences (e.g. Reis and Snow, 2001) and drawing dreams on waking has been used with Vietnam veterans experiencing PTSD (Morgan and Johnson, 1995) in order to help them process traumatic dream imagery, which reduced both the frequency and intensity of their nightmares. Second, people with ID frequently experience attention and memory deficits and as drawings provide an illustration of the images discussed, they can aid attention, information processing and retention (e.g. Clements, 1992).

In our adapted protocol, we are quite specific in our instructions. We ask our clients to change the ending of the dream so that they are rescued from the traumatic event by a strong and reliable force or person. We concentrate on them feeling safe, supported and protected and sure in the knowledge that the person who caused the trauma has been prevented from causing any further harm. The box below contains a brief description of one of the IRT interventions reported by Stenfert Kroese and Thomas (2006) as a way of illustrating this adapted IRT procedure.

Ms J, a 24-year old woman with Down's syndrome, reported typical PTSD symptoms that included flashbacks, nightmares (which occurred approximately three times a week), sleep disturbance, general anxiety, and a fear of the dark and of being alone. She stated that in the nightmares she relived a serious sexual assault that had occurred a year previously. Using IRT, the nature and cause of PTSD nightmares were explained and discussed and it was stressed that this technique would allow her to have more control over the nightmares. A 'new dream' was constructed collaboratively by drawing the scenario and then introducing a 'better ending' to the dream.

Ms J was asked how she wanted to be rescued from the perpetrator before the assault took place. She chose to call upon a fleet of police cars that drew up with sirens screaming and blue lights flashing before the sexual assault could take place. In her new version, the police locked the perpetrator in a cage with metal bars and drove him to the police station. Meanwhile, her mother arrived on the scene with a blanket and a thermos flask with hot tea, she was comforted and driven to her safe, comfortable home.

Ms J was conscientious in rehearsing this new dream before bedtime and combined the rehearsal with a relaxing routine: she would have a bath, carry out a simple relaxation exercise and then, with her mother's help, rehearse the new dream. After three fortnightly sessions, Ms J reported that the nightmares had ceased to occur. At 3 and 6 months of follow-up, this improvement had been maintained.

Figure 14.1: Case example of IRT

We make sure that this changing-the-dream technique always involves the introduction of visually striking characters and/or forces. The characters may be fictional and the forces magical as long as they have some significance for the client and we encourage our clients to choose these allies themselves rather than have them presented by the therapist. In the course of our clinical practice, we have worked with a wide variety of powerful and effective images. They include Arnold Schwarzenegger, the Pope, a porcelain fairy (placed beside the bed), strong/trustworthy family members, the power to fly through walls, and the power to see round corners. For some clients it has been difficult to report the content of their nightmares. One young woman needed to walk in the fresh air whilst talking about her dreams in order to combat nausea. It is important to stress (a, perhaps obvious, point) that IRT should only be carried out if the client is no longer in any danger. As the technique stresses having control over one's safety, it is essential that the client's home life is stable and without danger.

Like Krakow *et al.* (2001) and Willner (2004), we have found that IRT can also have a beneficial effect on other parts of our clients' lives. Being successful in dismissing past abusers who feature in the nightmares can give people confidence (and practice) to deal with unreasonable demands in their waking lives. Moreover, the exercise involves the therapist challenging 'powerless' and 'helpless' cognitions and generating 'in control', 'active' ones, which can be generalised to other situations.

Such small and uncontrolled studies, as the one described here, have shown promising results and suggest that adapted CBT techniques are well-tolerated and appreciated by our clients. But, as yet, we cannot draw firm conclusions regarding the effectiveness of TF-CBT as a treatment of PTSD in people with ID because large-scale, controlled studies are still lacking. What has been useful is that these case studies have taught us something about the modifications that are needed to accommodate differences and/or deficits in cognitive processing and verbal communication (e.g. Keesler, 2020).

Building on this small body of TF-CBT research, we (Stenfert Kroese *et al.*, 2016) developed a group therapy manual for people with ID using a CBT psycho-educational procedure to address the first stage of recovery from trauma (Herman, 1997; Courtois, 2004) and incorporating therapeutic methods that are routinely used to treat complex trauma in the general population. The manual was designed to provide survivors of trauma with a place to function in safe and trusting relationships, and increase their self-esteem and coping skills by promoting resilience, personal safety, self-care and emotion-regulation. The intervention we developed is also influenced by psychodynamic and feminist theories but it is mostly based on a TF-CBT model so that, throughout the programme, participants are helped to focus on and identify the impact of thoughts and other cognitive mediating events on their emotional state and behavioural responses.

The intervention is presented as a 'survivors' group and comprises a 12-week programme that includes:

1. agreement on group rules, group processes, focusing on confidentiality
2. development of an individual formulation
3. staying safe and stable
4. neuropsychology of trauma (how our bodies remember)
5. feelings and thoughts
6. understanding and managing emotions

7. improving relationships with others

8. depression and self-esteem

9. dissociation and different parts of ourselves

10. coping with triggers, memories, flashbacks and nightmares

11. self-harm and self-care

12. speaking up (assertiveness) and moving on (planning for the future).

Sessions typically include role-play and mindfulness or relaxation exercises, techniques designed to elicit and modify group members' cognitions and homework assignments, which, with their consent, are supported by support workers and carers who may also attend the group sessions.

We are influenced by the principles described by Holmes (2010) for effective group work and carefully prepare what may seem trivial aspects, such as the layout of the room, how our clients are welcomed into the building and the room in which the sessions take place, and the quality of the materials we use (including flipcharts, art materials, hand-outs, videos and beverages and biscuits provided during break times). We consider these to convey important messages, and to be essential for creating an environment where our clients can feel safe, valued, respected and listened to.

To find out if this TF-CBT group approach is effective, we carried out a small pilot study by collecting and collating outcome data for three therapy groups. Twelve people were recruited and their ages ranged from 21 to 46. Five of the group members chose to be accompanied by a support worker during the therapy sessions. We found that recruitment to the groups was unproblematic as referrers had become increasingly aware of the link between past trauma and current psychological problems, and the two local services where recruitment took place had developed trauma referral pathways that included the option of referral to TF-CBT groups.

Before the start of the group, all clients were seen individually and the specific traumatic events they had experienced were elicited using the Trauma Information form (Hall *et al.*, 2014). We made sure that none were in crisis or had recently experienced a placement breakdown, as we wanted to be sure that no one was suffering unsafe or unstable living conditions during the therapy. All had capacity to consent to the intervention and, with support, could complete the outcome measures.

During the one-to-one pre-group session, all clients completed the Impact of Event scale, a self-report measure of trauma that has been validated in a version adapted for people with ID (the revised Impact of Event scale ID (IES-ID); Hall *et al.*, 2014). Members also completed the Clinical Outcomes for Routine Evaluation – LD (CORE-LD) version (Marshall, Coiffait and Willoughby-Booth, 2013) and the Lancaster and Northgate Trauma scale (LANTS; Wigham *et al.*, 2014). The assessments were administered before the first group session and repeated within four weeks after the final session.

Ten participants completed the intervention and provided post-intervention outcome measures. Their median pre-treatment IES-ID score was well over twice the score reported by Hall, Jobson and Langdon (2014), which was to be expected as, although their sample had all experienced trauma, they had not been referred for treatment of PTSD. After completing the group, participants' scores decreased by a median of 27%, equivalent to a medium effect size. There were also small non-significant decreases post-treatment in median scores on the CORE-LD and LANTS and strong correlations between changes in IES-ID and CORE-LD and LANTS scores. We concluded from these quantitative data that TF-CBT as a group intervention for people with ID who present with complex PTSD has the potential to be an acceptable and feasible treatment.

To find out in detail how the members had experienced the group, five were interviewed individually. To aid their memory, a number of objects and illustrations that were used in the group sessions were presented. The semi-structured interview that we used was adapted from the interview used by MacMahon *et al.* (2015) and focused on members' expectations and experiences of the group, and perceived value and impact, if any, of taking part. The following questions were asked:

> *Try to remember back to before the group started. What did you think about joining the group?*
>
> *So now your group has finished, what do you think of the group?*
>
> *If you were in charge (the boss) of the group, what things would you change/keep the same?*
>
> *If someone you know was asked to take part in the next group, what would you say to them?*
>
> *If you were invited to a second group, what would you like to do in that group?*
>
> *Do you think that taking part in the group has made a difference to you?*
>
> *If I asked someone who knows you well (e.g. carer, partner) if you had changed at all since starting the group, what would they say?*
>
> *Can you think of anything else you would like to say about the group?*

Figure 14.2: Qualitative interview questions for group members

Several prompts were used if the participant struggled to answer the question. For example, for the first question the prompts were: 'What were you looking forward to in the group?' and 'Was there anything that made you feel worried or nervous before you started?'

Data were analysed according to interpretative phenomenological analysis (IPA) guidelines (Smith *et al.*, 2009) and the five themes that emerged were:

1. being listened to
2. it is nice to know you are not the only one
3. being in a group can be stressful
4. the importance of feeling safe
5. achieving and maintaining change.

The theme 'being listened to' has been reported by previous qualitative studies where participants with ID were asked to reflect on their experiences of individual or group therapy (Pert *et al.*, 2013; MacMahon *et al.*, 2015). Similar to these previous studies, our participants expressed surprise at being taken seriously and noted that the therapists valued their opinions and made an effort to understand their problems. The experience of being listened to and respected was compared with other settings in which they had felt ignored or dismissed. For example: 'I felt like an actual person who had the right to tell someone how he feels and not feel daft, because … at my place before … they were just sitting there like they weren't listening, because they'd turn their faces and I'd think "okay, you're not listening".'

Being in the presence of other people who had also experienced trauma was described as helpful although some members had initial misgivings about joining such a group: 'I was really nervous about meeting new people. My one problem is paranoia, so I thought everyone would judge me. But I got over it when I was there, after the first few I kept coming, and I could see we were all there for the same reason.'

The group members also talked about how being in a group can be stressful. There is a cost to being treated in a group as well as benefits. The cost, as experienced by one group member, was having to share the time and attention that the group therapists were able to devote to her: 'Sometimes it was quite difficult because when they [other group members] were anxious they obviously talk a lot (laughs) and so … staff were focusing all their attention on them and so we found it a bit difficult because obviously we couldn't really get a word in edgeways.'

Because of the trauma she had experienced in the past, one member did not enjoy the relaxation exercises that ended every group session, yet she endured this part of the session for the sake of the others: 'I know a lot of the people like the relaxation at the end but I didn't like it very much because I don't find it very easy to relax so when they were sat there with their eyes closed, I was thinking, "this is weird".'

Having a support person come with them worked well for a number of members who otherwise would not have attended the group sessions: 'If I'd gone on my own [without a support worker] then it wouldn't have worked. Certain things were hard to talk about'. But having support workers in the group can also have disadvantages: 'I didn't like the men in the group, the carers. They reminded me of the bad experiences I've had.' This group member found the presence of male support workers disturbing as male staff perpetrated the trauma she had experienced. As all service users who attended the groups had experienced severely traumatising events in their past, their evaluation of the group was often phrased in terms of how safe they felt in that setting.

One of the aspects of the group activities that the members remembered well and rated highly was the use of role-play. In our experience, role-play can make it easier to access cognitions and feelings, especially when the therapist takes the client's part and asks the client to 'direct the scene' and explain the incident in as much detail as possible. In group therapy, various group members and co-therapists can take on acting roles, be 'co-directors', 'producers' or 'stage hands' in order to involve everyone in the role-play. Seeing a therapist act out certain emotions is not only amusing for clients but can also make a lasting impression, which can normalise difficult feelings. Subsequently re-playing the scene, but with an agreed adaptive way of responding and with the main actor 'thinking aloud', can give insight into the cognitive model (illustrating that how we think can determine how we behave and feel) and the value of more functional ways of thinking and responding. These exercises were well-understood and remembered by our group members (e.g. '...role plays which was quite good. We did it in different ways, like in an aggressive way, or a calm way, and to see how people react when you do it in an aggressive or calm way') and, as in the MacMahon *et al.* (2015) study, staff taking part in the exercises appeared to be particularly memorable ('... and they (staff) joined in as well, which was good fun ... they're not sitting on it even though they're listening they're actually doing it with you, which was really great').

The group members that we interviewed made a number of clear and practical suggestions to improve the group intervention, which we have taken note of and incorporated into subsequent clinical practice. They include:

- avoid information overload: 'So if it was split up a bit and so you've got chance to sort of explain it, and sort of go through it, easily steps or baby steps for me would be a lot easier than too much information, it makes your head fried then.'
- more artwork and role-play: 'Bit more drawing and a bit more role-play, 'cause that was good.'
- provide an alternative to relaxation exercises: 'I know a lot of the people like the relaxation at the end but I didn't like it very much ... maybe some relaxing music of some sort.'
- more film: 'Maybe make some clips or something would be good, or DVDs, examples of people who have suffered.'
- more time: 'I'd like a bit more time. I'd like longer sessions and for the group to be over a longer time. So, just more of it really.'
- more information about how to cope with PTSD nightmares: 'And I'd like to do more about nightmares, to learn a bit more about that and how to cope with them.'

My own clinical experiences and the small, uncontrolled case and group studies that I have been involved in have made me confident that TF-CBT can be of benefit to clients with ID who suffer complex trauma symptoms. The evidence so far justifies, in my opinion, clinicians devoting their clinical time to adapting and applying TF-CBT for people with ID. But it has also become clear to me that we still need to spend more time and effort on developing the various adaptations that our clients require, and on proving that each of these has a valid function in their recovery process.

The future

The recent systematic review by Byrne (2020) shows that, at present, there is very little to choose between TF-CBT and EMDR in terms of effectiveness for PTSD symptoms. But they differ in the experiences offered to the client. TF-CBT is a highly verbal intervention that is designed to identify and modify over-interpretations of the actual levels of threat, and the beliefs and interpretations regarding the traumatic event. It is particularly suitable for addressing dysfunctional schema associated with PTSD, such as over-vigilance/inhibition and disconnection/rejection. By contrast, EMDR is traditionally less reliant on verbal expression and, because EMDR is a relatively short and simple procedure, and less reliant than CBT on verbal expression, it could be considered more suitable for people with ID. But we (Unwin *et al.,* 2019) have found that the standard EMDR protocol may be problematic. In our experience, clients find it difficult to understand the rationale and the terminology, the request for repeated self-report scores, and to manage the desensitization and reprocessing stages. We have found that to prevent dropout, clients need extensive preparation before starting EMDR so as to increase their engagement and to ensure that they have sufficient understanding of what they need to do and why. A group of clinicians and researchers (Willner *et al.,* 2018) have recently discussed these barriers and have come to the conclusion that the EMDR procedure can be made more accessible and acceptable by expanding the introductory psycho-educational phase using the techniques developed for our TF-CBT group work (Stenfert Kroese *et al.,* 2016), which allows the client to first benefit from psycho-education and stabilisation (PES) before undertaking the EMDR intervention.

We are currently involved in a four-year controlled trial led by Professor Paul Willner (Willner *et al.,* 2018), which uses a bespoke, simplified EMDR protocol preceded by a PES module. For the purposes of this trial, an introduction to bilateral stimulation has been added to the PES module and a modified EMDR protocol has been piloted. The major adaptations are:

1. making the stages, language and outcome measures more accessible
2. using 'tapping' instead of side-to-side finger movements as a form of bilateral stimulation
3. encouraging creative use of expression by using techniques from art and narrative therapy/storytelling (e.g. Lovett, 1999)

4. involvement of carers, where appropriate, to support the client within and/or between therapy sessions.

This national trial has been delayed by Covid-19 lockdown conditions and it is, as yet, too early to report on outcome data. However, we are excited about the prospect of collating the outcome measures of at least 144 adult clients, half of whom will be receiving an adapted PES plus EMDR protocol, which we anticipate will take up approximately 20 one-to-one sessions while the other half of the sample will receive treatment as usual. The study is designed as a randomised, controlled trial (RCT), with a nested qualitative study to assess fidelity, adherence and other factors that may potentially influence outcome. All participants will be followed up at four (after PES), eight (after EMDR) and 14 months. We hope that, as a first RCT in this area of clinical research, our findings may tell us whether our protocol has the potential to improve the mental health and quality of life of people with ID who suffer PTSD, whether it is cost-effective and whether the outcomes are influenced by the complexity of the PTSD presentation.

Conclusions

The number of published descriptive cases and small-scale quantitative and qualitative studies reporting on TF-CBT and EMDR interventions has recently grown and, taken together, represent a reasonably convincing case for clinicians to adopt a trauma-focused approach. There is a clear need for these types of interventions because (as argued above) our client group is particularly vulnerable to trauma and its long-term psychological consequences. In this chapter, I have considered the impact of trauma on our clients with ID, the main types of TF-CBT and the evidence for their effectiveness, before describing some examples of clinical work and attempts to report on the impact of trauma-focused interventions.

Although still at an early stage, advances have recently taken place in this clinically relevant research field. A number of assessment measures have been developed for PTSD, a small number of studies have studied the impact of trauma on people with ID and there is now a modest body of literature that has evaluated the effectiveness of CBT interventions for this client group. While these developments are promising, the field warrants more research and development, and we anticipate that better-controlled outcome data will become available in the next few years.

References

Baddeley A (1998) *Human Memory: theory and practice*. Needham Heights: Allyn and Bacon.

Barrowcliff AL, Oathamshaw SC & Evan C (2018) Psychometric properties of the Clinical Outcome Routine Evaluation Learning Disabilities-30 item (CORE-LD30). *Journal of Intellectual Disability Research* (62) 962–973.

Beadle-Brown J, Mansell J, Cambridge P, Milne A & Whelton B (2010) Adult protection of people with intellectual disabilities: Incidence, nature and responses. *Journal of Applied Research in Intellectual Disabilities* **23**, 573-584.

Beck AT, Rush AJ, Shaw BF & Emery G (1979) *Cognitive Therapy of Depression*. New York: Guilford Press.

Brewin CR, Andrews B & Valentine JD (2000) Meta-analysis of risk factors for post-traumatic stress disorder in trauma-exposed adults. *Journal of Consulting and Clinical Psychology* **68**, 748–766.

British Psychological Society (2018) *Positive Behaviour Support (PBS) – Committee and Working Group Position Statement*. BPS: Leicester: UK.

Byrne G (2018) Prevalence and psychological sequelae of sexual abuse among individuals with an intellectual disability: A review of the recent literature. *Journal of Intellectual Disabilities* **22**(3) 294–310.

Byrne G (2020) A systematic review of treatment for individuals with intellectual disability and trauma symptoms: A review of the recent literature. *Trauma, Violence, & Abuse*, https://doi.org/10.1177/1524838020960219.

Clements J (1992) *Severe Learning Disability and Psychological Handicap*. Chichester: Wiley.

Cohen JA, Mannarino AP & Murray LA (2011) Trauma-focused CBT for youth who experience ongoing trauma. *Child Abuse & Neglect* **35**, 637-646.

Costello H, Bouras N & Davies H (2007) The role of training community care staff awareness of mental health problems in people with intellectual disabilities. *Journal of Applied Research in Intellectual Disabilities* 2007 20 228–235.

Courtois CA (2004) Complex trauma, complex reactions: Assessment and treatment. *Psychotherapy: Theory, Research, Practice, Training* 41 (4), 412–425.

Daveney J, Hassiotis A, Katona C, Matcham F & Sen P (2019) Ascertainment and prevalence of post-traumatic stress disorder (PTSD) in people with intellectual disabilities. *Journal of Mental Health Research in Intellectual Disabilities* **12**(3-4), 211– 233.

Ehlers A & Clark DM (2000) A cognitive model of post-traumatic stress disorder. *Behaviour Research and Therapy* **38**, 319–345.

Engelhart I, van den Hout M & Smeets M (2011) Taxing working memory reduces vividness and emotionality of images about the Queen's Day tragedy. *Journal of Behavior Therapy and Experimental Psychiatry* (42) 32–37.

Emerson E & Brigham P (2014) Exposure of children with developmental delay to social determinants of poor health: cross-sectional case record review study. *Child: Care, Health and Development* **41**(2) 249-257.

Emerson E & Hatton C (2007) Mental health of children and adolescents with intellectual disabilities in Britain. *The British Journal of Psychiatry* **191** 493–499.

Ford JD, Courtois CA, Steele K, van der Hart O & Nijenhuis ERS (2005) Treatment of complex posttraumatic self-dysregulation. *Journal of Traumatic Stress* **18** 437-447.

Gilderthorp C (2015) Is EMDR an effective treatment for people diagnosed with both intellectual disability and post-traumatic stress disorder? *Journal of Intellectual Disabilities* **19** 58–68.

Hall J, Jobson L, & Langdon P (2014) Measuring symptoms of post-traumatic stress disorder in people with intellectual disabilities: the development and psychometric properties of the Impact of Event Scale – Intellectual Disabilities (IES-IDs). *British Journal of Clinical Psychology* **53** 315–332.

Herman JL (1997) *Trauma and Recovery*. New York: Basic Books.

Hulbert-Williams L, Hastings R, Owen DM et al (2014) Exposure to life events as a risk factor for psychological problems in adults with intellectual disabilities: a longitudinal design. *Journal of Intellectual Disability Research* **58**(1) 48–60.

Holmes G (2010) *Psychology in The Real World: Community-based groupwork*. Monmouth: PCCS Books.

Jahoda A, Stenfert Kroese B & Pert C (2017) *Cognitive Behaviour Therapy for People with Intellectual Disabilities – thinking creatively*. London: Palgrave McMillan.

Karatzias T, Shevlin M, Fyvie C, Hyland P, Efthymiadou E, Wilson D *et al.* (2017) Evidence of distinct profiles of posttraumatic stress disorder (PTSD) and complex posttraumatic stress disorder (CPTSD) based on the new ICD-11 Trauma Questionnaire (ICD-TQ). *Journal of Affective Disorders* **207** 181–7.

Keesler JM (2020) Trauma-specific treatment for individuals with intellectual and developmental disabilities: a review of the literature from 2008 to 2018. *Journal of Policy and Practice in Intellectual Disabilities* **17**(4) 332-345.

Krakow B, Hollifield M, Johnston L, Koss M, Schrader R, Warner TD, Tandberg D, Lauriells J, McBride L, Cutchen L, Cheng D, Emmons S, Germain A, Melendrez D, Sandoval D & Prince H (2001) Imagery rehearsal therapy for chronic nightmares in sexual assault survivors with posttraumatic stress disorder – a randomized controlled trial. *Journal of the American Medical Association* **286** 537–545.

Lovett J (1999) *Small Wonders: Healing childhood trauma with EMDR*. New York: Free Press.

McNally RJ & Shin LM (1995) Association of intelligence with severity of posttraumatic stress disorder symptoms in Vietnam combat veterans. *The American Journal of Psychiatry* **152**(6) 936–938.

MacMahon P, Stenfert Kroese B, Jahoda A, Stimpson A, Rose N, Rose J, Townson J, Hood K & Willner P (2015) 'It's made all of us bond since that course...' – a qualitative study of service users' experiences of a CBT anger management group intervention. *Journal of Intellectual Disability Research* **59**(4) 342-352.

Marshall K, Coiffait F-M & Willoughby-Booth S (2013) Assessing distress in people with intellectual disabilities. *Learning Disability Practice* **16** (3) 26-30.

Mason-Roberts S, Bradley A, Karatzias T, Brown M, Paterson D, Walley R, Truesdale M, Taggart L & Sirisena C (2018) Multiple traumatisation and subsequent psychopathology in people with intellectual disabilities and DSM-5 PTSD: a preliminary study. *Journal of Intellectual Disability Research* **62**(8) 730-736.

Mevissen L, Lievegoed R & De Jongh A (2011a) EMDR treatment in people with mild ID and PTSD: four cases. *Psychiatric Quarterly* **82**(1) 43–57.

Mevissen L, Lievegoed R, Seubert A & De Jongh A (2011b) Do persons with intellectual disability and limited verbal capacities respond to trauma treatment? *Journal of Intellectual and Developmental Disability* **36**(4), 278–283.

Mevissen L, Lievegoed R, Seubert A & De Jongh A (2012) Treatment of PTSD in people with severe intellectual disabilities: A case series. *Developmental Neurorehabilitation* **15**(3), 223–232.

Mevissen L, Didden R, Korzilius H & De Jongh A (2017) Eye movement desensitisation and reprocessing therapy for posttraumatic stress disorder in a child and an adolescent with mild to borderline intellectual disability: A multiple baseline across subjects study. *Journal of Applied Research in Intellectual Disabilities* **30** (1) 34–41.

Mitchell A, Clegg J & Furniss F (2006) Exploring the meaning of trauma with adults with intellectual disabilities. *Journal of Applied Research in Intellectual Disabilities* **19** 131–142.

Morgan CA & Johnson DR (1995) Use of a drawing task in the treatment of nightmares in combat-related post-traumatic stress disorder. *Art Therapy* **12** 244–247.

Morris JD, Webb EL, Parmar E, Trundle G & McLean A (2020) Troubled beginnings: the adverse childhood experiences and placement histories of a detained adolescent population with developmental disorders. *Journal of Advances in Mental Health and Intellectual Disabilities* **14**(6) 181–197.

Murray LK, Cohen JA, Ellis BH & Mannarino AP (2008) Cognitive behavioral therapy for symptoms of trauma and traumatic grief in refugee youth. *Child and Adolescents Psychiatric Clinics of North America* **17** 585–604.

Pert C, Jahoda A, Stenfert Kroese B, Trower P, Dagnan D & Selkirk M (2013) Cognitive behavioural therapy from the perspective of clients with mild intellectual disabilities: a qualitative investigation of process issues. *Journal of Intellectual Disability Research* **57**(4) 359–369.

Reis P & Snow S (2001) *The Dreaming Way: Dreamwork and Art for Remembering and Recovery*. Wilmette, IL: Chiron Publications.

Rose N, Kent S & Rose J (2012) Health professionals' attitudes and emotions towards working with adults with intellectual disability (ID) and mental ill health. *Journal of Intellectual Disability Research* **56** (9) 854–864.

Shapiro F (1999) Eye movement desensitization and reprocessing (EMDR) and the anxiety disorders: Clinical and research implications of an integrated psychotherapy treatment. *Journal of Anxiety Disorders* **13**, 35–67.

Shapiro F (2001) *Eye movement desensitization and reprocessing: Basic principles, protocols, and procedures* (2nd edition). New York: The Guilford Press.

Shapiro F (2007) EMDR and case conceptualization from an adaptive information processing perspective. In: F. Shapiro, L. Kaslow, A. Maxfield (eds.) *Handbook of EMDR and Family Therapy Processes* (pp3–34). Hoboken/New York: Wiley,

Steil R & Ehlers A (2000) Dysfunctional meaning of posttraumatic intrusions in chronic PTSD. *Behaviour Research and Therapy* **38** 537–558.

Stenfert Kroese B, Dewhurst D & Holmes G (2001) Diagnosis and drugs: help or hindrance when people with learning disabilities have psychological problems? *British Journal of Learning Disabilities* **29**(1) 26–33.

Stenfert Kroese B & Thomas G (2006) Treating chronic nightmares of sexual assault survivors with an intellectual disability – Two descriptive case studies. *Journal of Applied Research in Intellectual Disabilities* **19** (1) 75-80.

Stenfert Kroese B, Rose J, Heer K & O'Brien A (2013) Mental health services for adults with intellectual disabilities – what do service users and staff think of them? *Journal of Applied Research in Intellectual Disabilities* **26**(1) 3–13.

Stenfert Kroese B (2014) CBT with people with intellectual disabilities. In: A Whittington and N Grey (eds) *How to Become a More Effective CBT Therapist – Mastering Metacompetence in Clinical Practice*. Oxford: Wiley Blackwell.

Stenfert Kroese B, Jahoda A, Pert C, Trower P, Dagnan D & Selkirk M (2014) Staff expectations and views of cognitive behaviour therapy (CBT) for adults with intellectual disabilities. *Journal of Applied Research in Intellectual Disabilities* **27**(2) 145–153.

Stenfert Kroese B, Willott S, Taylor F, Smith P, Graham R, Rutter T, Stot A & Willner P (2016). Trauma-focussed cognitive behaviour therapy for people with mild intellectual disabilities: Outcomes of a pilot study. Advances in Mental Health and Intellectual Disabilities 10 299–310.

Tezel FK, Kislac ST & Boysan M (2015) Relationships between childhood traumatic experiences, early maladaptive schemas and interpersonal styles. *Archives of Neuropsychiatry* **52** (3) 226–232.

Truesdale M, Brown M, Taggart L, Bradley A, Paterson D, Sirisena C et al (2019) Trauma-informed care: a qualitative study exploring the views and experiences of professionals in specialist health services for adults with intellectual disabilities. *Journal of Applied Research in Intellectual Disabilities* **32** 1437–144.

Unwin G, Willott S, Hendrickson S & Stenfert Kroese B (2019) Eye movement desensitization and reprocessing for adults with intellectual disabilities: Process issues from an acceptability study. *Journal of Applied Research in Intellectual Disabilities* **32** (3) 635–647.

Vereenooghe L & Langdon P E (2013) Psychological therapies for people with intellectual disabilities: A systematic review and meta-analysis. *Research in Developmental Disabilities* **34** (11) 4085–4102.

Wigham S, Taylor JL & Hatton C (2014) A prospective study of the relationship between adverse life events and trauma in adults with mild to moderate intellectual disabilities. *Journal of Intellectual Disability Research* **58** (12) 1131–1140.

Willner P (2004) Brief cognitive therapy of nightmares and post-traumatic ruminations in a man with a learning disability. *British Journal of Clinical Psychology* **43** 459–464.

Willner P (2015) The neurobiology of aggression: implications for the pharmacotherapy of aggressive challenging behaviour by people with intellectual disabilities. *Journal of Intellectual Disability Research* **59** (1) 82–92.

Willner P & Lindsay WR (2016) Cognitive behavioral therapy. In: NN Singh (ed) *Handbook of Evidence-Based Practices in Intellectual and Developmental Disabilities* (pp283–310). New York: Springer.

Willner P (2018) Eye movement desensitisation and reprocessing for symptoms of post-traumatic stress disorder in adults with learning disabilities. *NIHR Health Technology Assessment Programme* 17/125

Young JE (1999) *Cognitive Therapy for Personality Disorders: A schema-focused approach.* Sarasota, FL: Professional Resource Press.

Chapter 15: Some concluding comments: acknowledge, identify and intervene

Allan Skelly

'Not everything that is faced can be changed.
But nothing can be changed until it is faced.'

– James Baldwin

We have established that intellectual disability (ID) is associated with increased exposure to adversity and, therefore, a heightened risk for psychological trauma. This book has not focused on physical trauma, and it could be said that this is a gap for other authors to fill. We have found that many people presenting with various forms of psychological distress to clinical settings will report physical effects of their historical maltreatment. This book addresses the unwanted and distressing effects of psychological trauma, which, of course, can follow a physical injury or condition. As suggested in the subtitle, we seek for this issue to be acknowledged, identified, and addressed through intervention. We are also interested in future directions.

Acknowledge

Emerson and Hatton (2007) estimated that 36% of children and adolescents with ID warranted a diagnosis of a 'psychiatric disorder'[3] compared to 8 per cent of children without an ID. Until relatively recently, only age, gender and level of disability were systematically researched as potential causal factors of high mental health diagnosis rates in people with ID (Enfield *et al.*, 2011). Hassiotis and

---

3   Diagnosis of mental disorder, as opposed to high levels of distress that require clinical help, is disputed by many psychologists and others on grounds of poor reliability and/or validity (you could easily get a different label from a different doctor) and conceptual convergence (diagnoses overlap, and several could be applied to your particular condition).

Turk (2012) found that level of intellectual impairment itself 'has a pathoplastic effect on psychopathology'. In contrast, Emerson and Hatton (2007) completed a comprehensive report that identified a broad range of risk factors associated with an ID, which might cause mental health problems in and of themselves. These included poor general health, greater exposure to adversity, having only one parent, living in poverty, conflict in the family, parental mental health problems, and fewer friends. The authors concluded that the concomitant mental health problems occurred 'simply because of their increased chances of being exposed to poverty, social exclusion and more challenging family environments'. While this helps avoid a fatalistic assumption that ID directly causes mental health problems, the report did not consider psychological trauma per se, and focuses on the need for intervention, which is primarily material, financial and focused on increased contact with peers.

Emerson *et al.* (2010) had found that parents of children with ID had higher rates of psychiatric diagnosis than parents of children without ID (thus raising risk of 'generational transmission' of forms of mental health issues), but these differences disappeared once socio-economic conditions were controlled in the data analysis. These authors actually suggested that socio-economic stress can even be a cause of cognitive impairment itself as well as being a result of caring for a child with ID.

We need to be very careful when a person is supported because they are considered to have 'challenging behaviour'. In considering the causes of behaviour that challenges, and its relationship to mental health disorders, Bowring *et al.* (2017) listed 'vulnerabilities' as biological (mobility, vision, epilepsy, autism, specific genetic syndromes) and psycho-social (communication issues, poor engagement, congregate care). In the resulting framework for understanding behaviour that challenges proposed by the authors, they list the impact of such behaviours as biological (effects of psychotropic medication, harm to self) and psychosocial (exclusion, harm to others, mental health issues).

This paper is quite typical of research that is associated with behavioural models, in that it does not mention trauma or attachment either as potential causal factors, or in terms of the traumatic effects of behaviours and their impact on close relationships. This is not only an issue in terms of lack of consideration of these factors. There are also issues in behavioural models of behaviours that challenge in locating the behaviour as belonging to an individual, with external factors acting on them (rather than being a function of human interactions within a system of attachment relationships). Often, professionals and carers will use 'challenging behaviour' as though it was a mental health diagnosis in comments such as 'he often has a behaviour', meaning there was a particular interaction that was difficult to manage or was seen as risky. Indeed, 'challenging behaviour' is a potential diagnosis using psychiatric classification, and can be made without reference to the past experience of the person at all.

Further, the concepts of behavioural theory are not very compatible with attachment theory. They cannot easily be bolted on to each other, and this can cause a failure to emphasise maintenance and continuation of attachment bonds as outcomes, as opposed to reductions in behaviours that challenge (which is itself not always achieved or maintained by behavioural methods) and environmental enhancement (which is also difficult to achieve).

One might have thought that the concept of challenging behaviour, which is socially defined in terms of its cultural abnormality, would take clear account of the weight of childhood experiences and the importance of early care relationships. Maybe, because the notion that childhood trauma is a cause of mental health problems is seen as reminiscent of Freud and psychoanalysis, it has been disavowed, or at least not emphasised in favour of the person's current conditioning in the here-and-now. The exception is where the person demonstrates flashbacks, or specific forms of cognitive or behavioural avoidance e.g. following a serious event, such as a car crash i.e. a specific behavioural treatment is required for a specific disorder, which is secondary to the primary behavioural treatment. It should be said that the group of people who would find flashbacks and cognitive avoidance most difficult to explain would be those with severe and profound intellectual disabilities, simply because of limited formal communication skills. This is precisely the group most likely to receive a behavioural treatment programme rather than the space and time of the psychotherapy room.

Since Felitti *et al.* (1998) illustrated the importance of adverse childhood experiences (ACEs) in determining health outcomes, trauma as a causal factor of distress has been much harder to ignore, though this remains a problem within ID services and policy. When trying to predict mental and behavioural distress, we must add the emphasis of the powerful impact of past and current maltreatment on health. Such experiences would seem to offer at least a partial explanation of these high rates in a significant proportion of those needing support with mental and behavioural distress. As seen in Chapter 6, high rates of neglect and abuse of people with ID seem to be endemic in liberal English-speaking democratic countries, although it would seem likely that a lack of epidemiological studies in other countries, rather than better treatment, are the reason for cross-cultural evidence. As the saying goes, absence of evidence is not evidence of absence.

This book tries to fill the gaps in awareness that appear to have developed for people with ID. In Chapter 2, Roger Wilczek offers the service-user perspective based on a semi-structured interview, but it is also so much more. I have had the privilege of working with Roger for several years in partnership to develop his role as an Expert by Experience. This chapter escapes theory and third-party comment; it is an articulate expression of what it is like to grow up with being devalued in the eyes of others, and subjected to repeated, and often systematic abuse. In identifying the denigrated terms with which others defined him, like "spacca", "loser" and "dipshit", Roger's chapter illustrates how trauma changes the very essence of personality when it occurs early in development; that education can be nightmarish; adult life lonely and unsafe; and how the appropriate care fails to be offered. The effects on self-esteem, self-worth and psychological state are clearly communicated; Roger's gift is to cut straight through to the essence of what needs to change, that a disability does not make us less deserving of love. I would only add that it is never too late to address this, and that unconditional love itself can be a basis of intervention, a neglected pillar of care policy.

Valerie Sinason (Chapter 3) and others have for some time pointed out the tendency for people with ID to be a low priority in the minds of those who seek to address mental distress and posited that this has been largely an unconscious process. It had not been faced. It may still not be faced – and what must be faced includes exclusion, cruelty, and an 'unoffered chair' (Bender, 1993). Historically, there was very little access to talking therapies, despite many people being shown to do very well when it is offered (e.g. Shepherd and Beail, 2017; Vereenooghe and Langdon, 2013; Skelly et al., 2018).

I have tried to link this lack of mentalisation of the plight of people with ID to the historical preference for institutionalisation and operant conditioning models of care (Skelly, 2019). Despite the conscious intention to add social value and ensure the well-being of people with intellectual disabilities, this culture contained the seeds of exclusion, coercion, punitive treatments, and, tragically, a disdain for the necessity of close loving bonds from caregiving adults, which has had a profound and lasting impact on the policy and research focus for people with ID. Now in the 2020s, there is no UK government policy document that explicitly addresses the need to prioritise placement permanence, close and loving relationships, and enhancements to care arrangements that can meet the attachment needs of children with ID. This is in sharp contrast to children who are at risk of going into the formal care system, who have a dedicated set of national clinical guidelines entitled Children's Attachment (National Institute for Clinical and Care Excellence, 2015, NG 26). The irony that children with ID are over-represented in this group, but explicitly excluded as a subject of the guideline, appears to confirm that awareness of their predicament is suppressed or avoided not only at the level of individuals but also at the level of societal priorities - specifically, in the policy objectives of health and social care bodies.

As pointed out by Nigel Beail (Chapter 4), models of trauma can be limiting in themselves. I am perennially perplexed that Freud's idea of trauma, which is clearly so influential and the basis of so much contemporary understanding of trauma, is not more explicitly adopted. Perhaps this should not be surprising, given that he disavowed the high rates of sexual abuse in his initial group of patients, on the grounds that it seemed almost impossible that it could be true, and must be a common fantasy in people with severe mental distress (letter to Fliess, 21 September, 1887). But the mechanised destruction of the First World War made the effect of actual adversity impossible to ignore, since many shell-shocked soldiers developed medically unexplained symptoms that responded very often to the talking-cure approach.

Consider Freud's definition:

"[Trauma can be defined as] any excitations from the outside which are powerful enough to break through the protective shield; there is no longer any possibility of preventing the mental apparatus from being flooded with large amounts stimulus that which have broken in; and binding of them.'

– Freud, 1920, Beyond the Pleasure Principle

He later added the feature of helplessness to this definition. Nigel Beail's assertion in Chapter 1 that we need to incorporate a developmental perspective, rather than just more widespread use of post-traumatic stress, can be seen as an allusion to the point that Freud makes about 'unwanted binding'; trauma fundamentally attaches itself to one's memory, one's emotions, one's very physiology. This should never be minimised or denied. In Chapter 1 Nigel also alludes to the power threat meaning framework, which emphasises what actually happened to a person, and how any mental health issues would reflect this. This is an important approach, because, unlike the concept of mental disorder, it starts from the assumption that traumatic reactions are continuing reasonable responses to unreasonable events. It is not a matter of simply realising that the threat has gone. It has remained as an 'object' or an attachment in the mind, and needs to be managed by the mind. Apt then, that Freud would have said that the ego, the very seat of reason, is vanquished by trauma, leaving one's mental life in a frightening state where one can no longer actually tell how much threat is actually present. We are likely to need help to see trauma for what it is, because our reason alone cannot remove its effect.

Identify

Since safeguarding procedures in the care sector are now well-established, there should be widespread knowledge of what to do when we notice that someone in our care may have been maltreated. If those involved acknowledge the ubiquity and centrality of trauma-informed care (TIC), at the level of the everyday care environment, it is essentially a matter of training at all levels, as has been modelled by NHS Education for Scotland for the public sector across that country, following incorporation of TIC into public policy. This lead taken by the Scottish Government and its agencies is to be recommended in all jurisdictions.

Where there is access to professional support, it is not actually that hard for clinical staff to identify trauma in people with ID who may present with severe and/or enduring distress to clinical services. Routine enquiry, using clinical interview or a simplified version of the adverse childhood experience (ACE) checklist, is a straightforward addition to the assessments that community learning disability services can offer. There are also measures that can screen for traumatic reactions (such as the LANTS) or attachment difficulties (MAS-T, QuERRS). The issue with identification is mainly a lack of policy direction, as the tools are available (see Chapter 6). This means that all that is required in terms of identification is:

- a raising of awareness among all health and social care professionals, or preferably the entire public and care sectors
- routine enquiry in primary care settings into adverse experiences
- dissemination of the appropriate screening tools to suitably skilled community teams to detect traumatic effects of adversity
- for carers, access to awareness training, specialised support
- clear routes to specialised therapies for the most severely traumatised people
- incorporation of TIC into the centre of the public policy narrative, as has already happened in Scotland.

Pat Frankish (Chapter 5) proposes a model of inevitable developmental trauma varying only by degree, which an ID makes more marked, and contests that this idea has been resisted because it is very painful to think about. The Frankish model is based on the separation-individuation theory of Margaret Mahler, who identified stages of emotional development, which diverges from skills development (adaptive behaviour) and intellectual or cognitive functioning. People will hopefully progress from a symbiotic relationship to their carer, to differentiation, through practicing, rapprochement, and, finally, individuation. An important idea in this approach is that 'double trauma' has more profound effects the earlier it occurs in development. The earlier it occurs, the more it impacts upon the person's sense of self, which can become a state of constant response to trauma, coming to be seen as 'severe challenging behaviour'; even, as a case where difficulties seem intractable, unresponsive to behavioural and pharmacological interventions, but where there is clearly some urgency and a need to develop some kind of safe haven.

Intervene

In terms of intervention, we have seen a number of approaches presented in this book. Elizabeth Goad (Chapter 7) demonstrates how principles developed from both the attachment theory and compassion-focused theory of Paul Gilbert can actually alter the very structures, pathways and narratives of community learning disability services, but with a welcome practical focus that will be able to manage resistance, and influence other important partners for these teams.

Despite my comments above, Cathy Harding (Chapter 8) is optimistic about change within positive behaviour support (PBS). Cathy suggests that relational outcomes can be incorporated into PBS, making changes such as identifying losses of care staff and sudden admissions as re-traumatising events rather than assuming these will be opportunities or emotionally neutral, and using Hughes' concept of blocked care, involving the entire support network in these discussions. This is an important note of hope, as PBS has achieved a privileged position in policy and procedure in health and social care settings, though I would argue that it needs fundamental reform and acceptance of TIC by its key advocates. The British Institute for people with Learning Disabilities (BILD) are making great strides in this area.

Intensive Interaction as presented by Judith Samuel and Sophie Doswell (Chapter 9) is an approach to communication for people with ID who may have very limited formal communication skills, and make their needs known through interaction with people who know them well. The parallels with attachment theory are very obvious, given that those who use intensive interaction are present, responsive, supportive of exploration, and comforting and helpful at times of distress or discomfort. However, carers may be dealing with past traumas that the person has no formal concept of, instead representing this in bodily responses or attachment insecurity or disorganisation. We could consider that intensive interaction is actually the form that psychotherapy should take for people without formal language skills, as, developmentally, this would be an analogue of very early parental care. This may raise issues about the intensity of support required to overcome trauma, and it will be complicated by issues such as chronic postural issues, physical pains and, potentially, increased loss of function across the lifespan.

We are offered another framework for clinical intervention in the form of dyadic developmental psychotherapy (DPP) by Nic Jones (Chapter 10). As with Elizabeth Goad's approach, Nic is keen for the principles to be widened to service-level or organisational interventions, rather than merely an approach to psychological therapy. Given that DPP draws on attachment theory, DPP will have a strong emphasis on the caregiver relationship and working to strengthen this by supporting resilient connections that can overcome blocked care. Through case examples, it is shown how DPP can address cases that have not been successfully treated within a PBS pathway prior to applying DPP.

Nigel Beail has long been an advocate for psychotherapy access for people with ID. In Chapter 11, he presents us with an overview of trauma-informed psychodynamic therapy based on Freud's early work, which is starting to show a promising evidence base, illustrating that the unoffered chair may well have been needless discrimination. Nigel offers case examples to demonstrate how trauma can be addressed within psychotherapy sessions.

The Frankish approach to intervention (Chapter 12) offers a very practical method of identifying the dominant stage, approaching the person with caregiving behaviours appropriate to that stage, and measuring change towards the next stage. While this is actually a discrete conceptual model, there are clearly parallels and compatibility with attachment theory, although this model may offer additional adjustments according to the person's assessed level of emotional development. Importantly, it may be possible to offer this therapy to people with very limited communicative functioning and address the 'unoffered chair' for the most vulnerable people with the least practical independence. This approach is intended to be followed easily by caregivers with no prior training in psychodynamic concepts, and to be easily added to behavioural support plans so as to provide a holistic method of intervention primarily informed by emotional development.

Brett Kahr (Chapter 13) also offers a psychodynamic understanding, but this time through his work with forensic patients, who are seen because of the risk they present to others. Brett takes us right back to Freud's original thoughts about the talking cure, in the process demonstrating how in his own work with those who are both vulnerable and threatening, 'insults' can replace 'spears', and therefore address this risk by a process of shared understanding.

Clearly this book has explored the strong tradition of psychodynamic theory, and its derivatives in conceptualising trauma, and how it should be addressed. However, it is important to consider work inspired by other theoretical traditions. In Chapter 14, Biza Kroese describes the application of adapted cognitive behavioural therapy (CBT) based interventions for the symptoms associated with diagnosis of post-traumatic stress disorder (PTSD) and the development of trauma-focused CBT (TF-CBT). For many people, a symptomatic approach will be very helpful and the evidence is beginning to accrue. Again, case examples are given to illustrate how the model can be helpful. I noted that the three-stage model described aims to achieve stabilisation, reworking of meaning of the trauma, and finally trust in others and the world. This resonates with the idea of safe-haven from attachment theory, and reminds me that a secure emotional base in the mind can arise from the repeated offer of such a haven in the person's experience of the mind of their therapist. I am hopeful that colleagues who use CBT can gain something from the models that focus more heavily on empathy and/or mentalisation in the re-working of trauma, and acknowledge the personal factors brought by the therapist that will make change happen through their positive attachment bond to their patient.

Also highly relevant to trauma work is the field of eye movement desensitisation and reprocessing, or EMDR, which is also described in Chapter 14. Some may disagree with its originators as to the ingredients of the therapy that actively make for change, and others may find the bilateral stimulation (left-right alternated optical attention) to lack credibility. Yet there can be no doubt that this approach is promising in its results with those who receive a PTSD diagnosis. However, since the 'body keeps the score' with trauma, it may well be that EMDR indeed has some physiological basis. To my mind, the main barrier might be the person's ability to follow instructions, so for people with more severe ID, perhaps intensive interaction or a more non-directive approach will be more suitable.

Future directions

In terms of future directions for study and thought, we no longer require evidence that trauma is visited on people with ID more than on others, despite their pre-existing vulnerability. This is a continuing moral outrage, as this has not resulted in anything like sufficient policy priority for this group. We cannot overstate how strongly we wish to make this point.

We can be reasonably confident that people with mild to moderate ID presenting with psychological distress – traditionally considered as anger, depression, or anxiety – can benefit from psychological therapies and these should be made available. Requiring a 'special' evidence base for people with ID before offering them the same treatments as everyone else smacks of discrimination. This may well be unwitting and unintentional, but the question needs to be asked as to why the assumption is made (that they will not work) in the absence of positive evidence showing their ineffectiveness.

It is imperative for clinical researchers to investigate the approaches explored in this book further. A randomised controlled trial (RCT) – the 'gold-standard' expected for a psychological approach to be considered to have positive evidence – is not beyond the abilities of several of our contributors and their colleagues. For example, an RCT for trauma-informed PBS, as it was described by Cathy Harding in Chapter 8, could be completed with offering every other referral the modified approach and then on achieving enough statistical power (numbers of cases), the results compared to those who receive 'standard' PBS. Of course, this entails careful thought to avoid disadvantaging anyone. For example, if clinicians feel obliged to offer the modified form of PBS to a particular subgroup in particular need, then randomisation may prevent some people from getting the right help at the right time. Another possibility is to simply consider those who have had 'failed' PBS and attempt the modified approach, to see if it fails a second time. There is already high-quality case-series evidence that adding attachment-based working to behaviour therapy for children with visual and severe intellectual disabilities can be more effective than behaviour therapy alone (Sterkenberg *et al.*, 2007).

We also know that approaching attachment directly can also be helpful for many people with mild to moderate ID receiving psychotherapy. Skelly and Burman (2015) noted that in 44 referrals for psychological therapy, quantified signs of preoccupied or disorganised attachment representations led to more sessions for those clients, although all clients improved after flexible-length therapy. However, as with CBT, we have yet to find out if psychodynamic therapy, such as that offered in that study, works because of improved attachment to the therapist, which leads to a reduction in distress, or if it is another factor or mix of factors – even placebo. This highlights the importance of well-designed efficacy studies – several forms of input are likely to make you feel better – but we still don't know exactly why. Yet this is not particular to people with ID; it is a question for all psychotherapies.

Those with avoidant attachment behavioural systems (those who were emotionally rejected as children) may need a lot of pre-engagement work as they will be expecting the care-giving system to reject them emotionally; those with preoccupied attachment (whose parents were intermittently available, ill or vacillating) may feel that they require therapy for years; and those with disorganised attachment may be terrified by the whole process, at least initially.

The other specialised forms of psychotherapy presented in this book need to develop beyond case studies (DDP and EMDR) and case series (disability psychodynamic psychotherapy), as methodologies are often weak, with small samples, fail to offer control groups or conditions, and use different assessment methods that are often non-standardised. On the other hand, all of the available evidence is at least supportive of the different approaches and, as has been said, there is almost no positive evidence of ineffectiveness.

Let us remember, though, that specialised therapies are only one aspect of TIC. We need to lobby on the basis of the increased exposure to adversity that people with ID are a priority, and they should never be left out of scope by national policy documents without a clear research basis for this (which seems to be unlikely in most instances).

One area for cross-fertilisation seems to be the relationship of separation-individuation theory to the empirical assessment of emotional development in the Netherlands (e.g. Sterkenburg *et al.,* 2021). These studies are interesting because they demonstrate that emotional development is quantitatively different from intellectual development, though related, and it may help us test the idea that trauma in early development causes unnecessary 'double trauma'.

Family carers and anyone working in a professional capacity with people with ID should have at least a basic awareness training in TIC, and professionals are likely to require more than this at some point in their care career. Therefore, we strongly recommend that the approach of the Scottish Government in its public sector education programme for TIC is adopted in all jurisdictions.

To end on a hugely important point: the person's voice – what they want to tell us – must become better known. It must be heard in the documents that describe them, in the conversations people have with them or about them, in their official records, in the way their support services are designed, and in the policies that exert power over them. We must remember that human beings do not talk about their lives in the abstract; it is the stuff of experience, of hurt, loss and joy, which cannot always be put into words. Where this is so, we should help them to do just that, even if we must co-create their story to bring it forth.

We know that they are owed this. This generation will not be forgiven by the judgement of history if we do not address trauma in the lives of people with ID. Preventing trauma by effective early intervention is only going to be achieved some of the time. However, it is clearly possible for trauma to heal. As with others who receive help, people with ID will find their way to memory, but only if they are given the chance.

References

Bender M (1993) The unoffered chair: the history of therapeutic disdain towards people with a learning difficulty. *Clinical Psychology Forum* **54** 7–12.

Bowring DL, Painter J & Hastings RP (2019) Prevalence of challenging behaviour in adults with intellectual disabilities, correlates, and association with mental health. *Current Developmental Disorders Reports* **6** (1) 173–181.

Enfield SL Ellis LA & Emerson E (2011) Comorbidity of intellectual disability and mental disorder in children and adolescents: A systematic review. *Journal of Intellectual & Developmental Disability* **36** (2) 137–143.

Emerson E & Hatton C (2007) *The Mental Health of Children and Adolescents with Learning Disabilities in Britain*. Lancaster, UK: Foundation for People with Learning Disabilities and Lancaster University.

Emerson E, Hatton C, Llewellyn G, Blacker, J & Graham H (2010) Socioeconomic position, household composition, health status and indicators of the well-being of mothers and children with and without intellectual disabilities. *Journal of Intellectual Disability Research* **50** (12) 862–873.

Felitti VJ, Anda RF, Nordenberg D, Williamson DF, Spitz AM, Edwards V & Marks JS (1998) Relationship of childhood abuse and household dysfunction to many of the leading causes of death in adults: The Adverse Childhood Experiences (ACE) Study. *American Journal of Preventative Medicine* **14** 245–258.

Hassiotis A & Turk V (2012) Mental health needs in adolescents with intellectual disabilities: Cross-sectional survey of a service sample. *Journal of Applied Research in Intellectual Disabilities* **25** 252–261.

National Institute for Health and Care Excellence (NICE, 2015) *Challenging Behaviour and Learning Disabilities: prevention and interventions for people with learning disabilities whose behaviour challenges* [online]. Available at: nice.org.uk/guidance/ng11.

Shepherd C & Beail N (2017) A systematic review of the effectiveness of psychoanalysis, psychoanalytic and psychodynamic psychotherapy with adults with intellectual disability: Progress and challenges. *Psychoanalytic Psychotherapy* **31** 94–117.

Skelly A (2019) Historical myopia and behaviourism in clinical psychology. *Clinical Psychology Forum* **316** 32-35.

Skelly A & Burman H (2015) Clinician-rated attachment and outcome of psychodynamic psychotherapy for people with intellectual disabilities. *Bulletin of the Faculty for People with Intellectual Disabilities of the British Psychological Society* Vol. 13 (1) 20–30.

Skelly A, McGeehan C & Usher R (2018) An open trial of psychodynamic psychotherapy for people with mild-moderate intellectual disabilities with waiting list and follow up control. *Advances in Mental Health and Intellectual Disabilities* **12** (5/6) 153–162.

Sterkenburg P S, Janssen CGC & Schuengel C. (2007) The effect of an Attachment based behaviour therapy for children with visual and severe intellectual disabilities. *Journal of Applied Research in Intellectual Disabilities* **21** 2 126–135.

Sterkenburg PS, Kempelmann GEM, Hentrich J, Vonk J, Zaal S, Erlewein R & Hudson M (2021) Scale of emotional development – short: reliability and validity in two samples of children with an intellectual disability. *Research in Developmental Disabilities* **108** 103821.

Vereenooghe L & Langdon PE (2013) Psychological therapies for people who have intellectual disabilities: A systematic review and meta-analysis. *Research in Developmental Disabilities* **34** 4085-4102.

Other titles from Pavilion Publishing

Frankish Assessment of the Impact of Trauma in Intellectual Disability (FAIT)
by Dr Pat Frankish (2019)

The CaPDID Training Manual. A Trauma-informed Approach to Caring for People with a Personality Disorder and an Intellectual Disability
by Jo Anderson, Dr Max Pickard, Emma Young and Toby Young (2020)

Trauma-informed Care in Intellectual Disability. A self-study guide for health and social care support staff
by Dr Pat Frankish (2019)

Nought to three – becoming me. A guide for parents (and those who support them)
by Dr Pat Frankish (2019)

Mental Health in Intellectual Disabilities (5th Edition)
by Dr Colin Hemmings (2018)

Guided Self-help for People with Intellectual Disabilities and Anxiety and Depression
by Eddie Chaplin (Ed) (2014)

Introduction to Mental Health and Mental Wellbeing for Staff Supporting Adults with Intellectual Disabilities
by Eddie Chaplin, Karina Marshall-Tate, Steve Hardy and Ruwani Ampegama (2019)

Introduction to Mental Health and Mental Wellbeing for staff supporting adults with intellectual disabilities: a training pack
by Ruwani Ampegama, Karina Marshall-Tate, Eddie Chaplin and Steve Hardy (2019)

Moss-PAS (ID), Moss-PAS ChA, Moss-PAS Diag(ID), Moss-PAS Check. Mental health assessments for adults and children with and without intellectual disabilities
by Dr Steve Moss

I Can Feel Good. DBT-informed skills training for people with intellectual disabilities and problems managing emotions (2nd Edition)
by Sarah Ashworth, Natalie Brotherton, Bridget Ingamells and Catrin Morrisey (2019)

Attachment-based Practice with Adults. Understanding strategies and promoting positive change
by Clark Baim and Tony Morrison (2011)